THE
RELUCTANT
YOGI

A Quirky Guide to the
Practice that Can
Change Your Life

Carla McKay

GIBSON SQUARE

Contents

Foreword

The ancient practice of yoga has been embraced by celebrities, new-age nuts and skinny fashionistas as a hip tool for modern living. Like any other trend with money-making potential, a whole raft of self appointed gurus have, over the years, soon arrived on the yoga scene, turning themselves into yoga brands complete with multi-media spin-offs, book deals, fashion lines and franchises.

Of course there are many devotees who regard yoga as an enjoyable physical, mental and spiritual discipline. But then there are some who think that, as with vanilla ice cream, you can just add in your favourite sauce. Feel like saying the Lord's Prayer while you're in Downward Dog? Try Christian yoga. Want to ogle others doing Downward Dog? Nude yoga might be for you. Fancy taking your own pet along to demonstrate Downward Dog? Doga (yoga for dogs) is coming to somewhere near you soon.

All of this is sad because, as I have discovered, later rather than sooner in my life, yoga in the traditional sense is for everyone, whatever their age, build or fitness level. In fact, the very people who would benefit from it the most, are likely to be those who are most put off by the flim flam surrounding the yoga world, as

I was for many years. This book is an attempt to redress the balance, to investigate what yoga is really all about, and to assess, without fear or favour, what it has to offer.

It is also the story of my own conversion from someone who scoffed at the very idea of yoga to someone who tries to get everyone she meets, from the boiler repair man to the chairman of the board, to give it a go.

Introduction

Do Not Attempt This at Home

It's early days in the quest for eternal youth: I have been to my first yoga class and am lying face down on the sitting room carpet, arms outstretched with one leg tucked awkwardly under my torso in what I fondly imagine to be the 'pigeon pose', apparently good for opening one's hips. I hadn't realised mine were closed till earlier that day.

The dogs are licking my face trying to revive me when my daughter walks in and screams: 'Mum, what happened?' I realise that from above, it probably looks as though a truck has run over me. Lesson One has been learned: never practise yoga in a room accessible to either other people or dogs.

Everybody was doing yoga; not just celebs with Gucci yoga mats (though they were much in evidence), but ordinary, quite rational people in the English countryside. It was said that yoga could change your life – and boy, did mine need changing.

That year I had separated from my husband, for reasons that were everything to do with me, and had moved out of our shared Oxfordshire house into a small cottage in the same village. A cottage I then shared with my 16-year-old son, whose sweet nature was being severely tested by adolescence, and my 14 year old daughter who was just embarking on a colourful career of getting expelled from every school she went. Oh, and I was reaching an age where I could barely conceal my panic about aging and see every wrinkle grow.

Yoga was widely reported at this time to be transformative in every area of life: physical, mental and spiritual. Everyone agreed it was the thing to do. Even the dogs did it every morning when they woke up, admittedly confining it to the one pose they knew – Downward Dog. All the buzz about yoga made me mutinous though. I could probably hack the poses (I had been good at gym in the dark ages), but I was definitely not going to chant Om or step reverentially into any room reeking of incense and decked out with Tibetan prayer flags. That kind of paraphernalia I associated with believers, with disciples, with bird-brained gullible fools who turned into Buddhists seconds after disembarking from the plane at Mumbai. Fatally, having been to the one class in the village hall, I put off going to another for a few years. It took that long to wear down my prejudice.

When I was growing up, no-one in the UK had really heard of yoga. It was at least a decade before middle-class kids trailed off to the East to find themselves. Physical exercise was pretty well confined to team sports and what used to be called 'physical jerks'*, both of them optimally performed in the freezing cold. At the school I went to, we ran round muddy fields wielding hockey sticks (or, worse, lacrosse sticks) in raw chapped hands. My fingers were additionally blown up with a vicious kind of chilblain owing to poor circulation, their tips numb and white. It was torture. I infinitely preferred being inside the relatively less arctic gymnasium where we sprang over the horse in double woofs and hung from the wall bars. In those days I could shin up a rope like a monkey and hang nonchalantly upside down – a skill I now seem to have lost, alas, although it hasn't been put to the test lately.

Then there was PT or PE at school sandwiched between double biology and maths which was something to be excused from (girls always had an excuse) at all costs. It could take almost any form, from what used to be called Swedish Gymnastics – a form of freestanding exercises involving flexions and extensions of the major joints of the body – to something even more gruesome that became popular in the 1960s, interpretative dance, in which you glided or galloped around the gym pretending to be flowers, or the wind, or a gazelle. After school it was of course up to you, and most people I knew never took any more strenuous exercise than raising a glass.

Nonetheless, people started to get serious about 'working out'. Many of the trends in exercise since the sixties seem to have been triggered by books. Dr Kenneth H. Cooper's groundbreaking book *Aerobics* was published in 1968, spawning a whole generation

obsessed with cardio-vascular fitness; then came Jim
Fixx's *The Complete Book of Running in 1977* – the best
selling non-fiction hardcover book ever – which gave
rise to the global phenomenon of jogging. It took a bit
of a knock when Jim Fixx, a formerly overweight magazine editor, was found dead by the side of a road in the
New England countryside aged only 52. He had suffered a massive heart attack in the middle of a run. Yet,
still people gallop, or more often shuffle on, and everyone from the nerd next door to world class eaters and
party-goers like Oprah, Gordon Ramsey and Puff
Daddy take part in marathons.

Yoga interest dates from the same time. It was in
1966, earlier than either of those, that B.K.S. Iyengar
published his international bestseller *Light on Yoga*
which renewed interest in yoga in the West, and
remains the gold standard reference book for practitioners of Hatha yoga for its illustration and explana-
tion of hundreds of asanas (yoga poses). Iyengar originally took up yoga to try to improve his poor health.
His mother had given birth to him during a flu epidemic leaving him sickly and weak and she later suc-
cumbed to malaria, TB and typhoid. Eventually he
became a yoga teacher in Pune, India, but it was a
meeting with the violinist Yehudi Menuhin, who
became his pupil, that led to international recognition.
Menuhin wrote the foreword to *Light on Yoga* in which
he says: 'The practice of yoga over the past 15 years has
convinced me that most of our fundamental attitudes
to life have their physical counterparts in the

body…'And of Iyengar he remarked: 'He is my master and my Guru… ever since I became his pupil and followed his course of exercises, I have not had any drug or medicine to cure any illness. I would trust him completely with my sons on top of a mountain in a thunderstorm, and know that he would bring them back unharmed.' Now, that's what I call a testimonial.

Light on Yoga undoubtedly played a large part in the popularisation of yoga outside India – especially hatha yoga of which Iyengar yoga is a form, known for its use of props such as blocks and belts as aids in performing asanas – but yoga is not a fad or a trend like 'dance aerobics' or 'step aerobics', neither is it a religion or a cult. It's a philosophy which has evolved over thousands of years which strives for mental, physical and spiritual balance.

Unfortunately, as far as I was concerned, it had been hijacked by the very people I tried to avoid ever reading about: Madonna, Gwynneth Paltrow and a whole lot of other celebri-yogis. Although, it has to be said that at least Gwynneth can quote passages from the *Yoga Sutras* in fluent Sanskrit, which gives her some yogini-cred in my book.

And, in any case, it wasn't just some quick-fix weight loss exercise I was after – it was youth; it was about halting the decline, turning back the clock, regaining lost strength and vitality. I knew people of my age who ran their socks off on treadmills or who tried every diet and exercise fad there was – and they still looked 100. These supermodels who posed on every cover with

their legs in impossible positions were already blessed
with youth, possibly eternal youth, goddamit. No, I
thought, I am not going to join the gang of golden-
limbed teeny weeny spandex wearing, mat-bag dan-
gling, organic chomping goddesses; there's got to be
another way for proper people like me who age normally, who drink, maybe even smoke, and who don't
have inviting yoga studios in their houses. And so, once
again, I put off changing my life.

---

* Physical jerks, (admirably described by George Orwell in *1984*) were a
series of regimented exercises, often commenced with an ear-splitting
whistle, and designed to cause maximum discomfort in the exerciser. If
you google the phrase now, most entries will tell you that Physical Jerks is
the name of a ska band.

1

Taking the Plunge

Having done enough research to get an A level in yoga studies, I saved up and finally decided to jump in the deep end and go straight off to India in search of yogic enlightenment. January had been horrible, as usual, and towards the end of the month, I was reunited with a long-lost cousin who was physically in pretty bad shape owing to liver disease. She was due to take a course of interferon to try to treat her Hepatitis C but wanted a restorative holiday in which to build up her immune system as best she could before the treatment started. She had heard that Indian Ayurvedic medicine was extremely beneficial and, like me, thought she wanted to try out yoga.

This seemed to be a sign. Wasting no time, I quickly searched on the internet for Ayurvedic treatment plus yoga and came up with a retreat in the mountains of Tamil Nadu above the once British hill station of Conoor in south-eastern India. It looked lovely – accommodation being in round 'glass cottages' set at intervals in the middle of a tea plantation stretching for miles in the blue distance. I liked the fact too that it billed itself as an Ayurveda & Yoga Retreat Hospital with a resident physician who would be on hand if my cousin's health took a turn for the worse. And, best of all, it was cheap compared to everything else on offer. In addition to yoga and meditation, the speciality programmes on offer were tantalising too: 'weight loss, total detoxification, anti-aging, stress, de-addiction, energy & strength, depression, sleep & diet, etc'. Obviously, I wanted and needed all of those things, so it was tricky just picking one. With enormous difficulty I plumped for weight loss as my primary aim.

I arrived at the retreat late one night in February having flown to Bombay, caught a connecting flight to Coimbatore, and then endured a hair-raising journey by car up twisting mountain lanes largely on the wrong side of the road. Unexpectedly, it was freezing cold. The owners had stayed up for me and I was led through a jungle path to my cottage where my cousin, Siobhan, had already been holed up for three days. 'She will not get out of her bed,' the owner told me. 'Not for yoga, not for massage, not for anything', she added.

I was too exhausted to tackle this one, and just fell straight into bed only to be woken what must have only been a couple of hours later by a banging at the door. A tiny Indian man stood there with a tray, on which were two dainty cups. I looked at my watch: 6 am – a tad early for my morning cup of tea, but still. Unable to see much in the gloom, I was just about to drink mine when Siobhan shrieked 'Don't touch it, they're trying to poison us.' I took a sip and spat it straight out – it was indeed filthy, but I doubted that it was lethal. It turned out this was the much lauded herbal concoction that was offered at sunrise every day for detoxing. Siobhan went back to sleep.

I dragged on some yoga clothes – the man told us the sunrise class was about to start in the yoga building – a circular building with a straw roof, wooden floor and a several large statuettes of Buddha, Krishna and other gods festooned with gaudy flowers. There were about ten other people already there, mostly youngish and mostly half asleep. Nobody spoke, thank goodness. A slim young man took us through some basic warm-up poses – mostly the sun salutation routine and, fittingly, the sun rose just as we were saluting it. I felt strangely positive about what lay ahead.

After the yoga, we spilled out onto a lawn as green and tended as an English vicarage garden where breakfast was served – a heavenly mix of fresh, tropical fruit and different, delicately scented and flavoured vegetable curries. Then it was time for our individual appointments with the resident Ayurvedic doctor.

Dr Mouli inspired confidence. A quiet, polite, bespectacled man, he first set about establishing my predominant mind/body type. According to Ayurvedic medicine, each of us has a unique mix of three doshas – or bodily humours – which make up our constitution. The word Ayurveda means 'science of life' and is the 5000 year old art of living in harmony with nature. The three doshas are Vata (space and air); Pitta (Fire and Water) and Kapha (Water and Earth). We all have in our make-up all three doshas but usually two are dominant and one is insignificant. There are various ways of ascertaining which dosha you are and Dr Mouli both studied my physical characteristics and asked a series of questions designed to establish my personality. At a grossly basic level, vata people are thin and nervous, pitta people are of medium build, pretty active and quick to anger, and kapha people are bigger, laid back and slow to anger. For the record, I was a pitta-vata, moderately active, moderately built and damn irritable. No surprise that I'm not a kapha person – whom Dr Mouli described as the 'earth mothers'.

For good health and well-being, he explained, the three doshas within a person need to be in balance according to your own original doshic make-up. In other words, it was important for me to maintain my pitta overload, followed by my sizeable vata character-istics and even my minimal kapha ones. This can be achieved by following particular lifestyle choices appro-priate to your dosha. What you eat, where you live, the work you do, the relationships you have and even just the passage of time can throw you into imbalance and if this is not corrected, you will have poor health.

On this basis, Dr Mouli prescribed a series of Ayurvedic massages for me, a particular (vegetarian of course) diet and special herbal medicines. This would all add up to the programme I was to follow that week. I couldn't wait.

The massages were a revelation. Nothing like the mamby-pamby, keep-your-knickers-on variety I had tried in health clubs in Europe. The massage room was dark, incense-filled and filled with fruity 'oms' coming from a speaker. Out of the gloom stepped two delicate girls of about twenty who asked me to strip off entirely and lie on a beautiful, oiled wooden table called a droni in Sanskrit. They then doused me liberally with a thick, nutty oil before simultaneously and in perfect harmony pummelling me to within an inch of my life. Did I say two delicate girls? I felt as though I had fallen into the hands of a bunch of navvies, so thoroughly was I squeezed, kneaded and rolled around. It was an extraordinary experience which left me feeling utterly wonderful and several pounds lighter.

Every day that week I had an Ayurvedic massage. Sometimes I was put into a hot steam capsule beforehand and sometimes the massage took the form of dripping oil onto my head. Each one was fabulous but none quite matched up to the thrashing I took the first time. The yoga classes – of which there were usually three a day – were also good. The teachers were always serious, silent young men who tailored the poses to their mostly western, mostly overweight and under stretched students. We did forward bends, downward dogs and lots and lots of sun salutations. I found these very difficult and marvelled at how some of the others (there were some student yoga teachers in the class too) could so effortlessly place their hands on the floor without bending their legs and then snake downwards and up into cobra in one fluid movement. But I learned a quick and important lesson during these classes: you get better the more you do it. At first, it's discouraging because you can only approximate the movement demonstrated. But gradually, you find you can do more and more.

Even Siobhan ventured out to some of the classes eventually and by the time she went home was a yoga convert. She had a lot of back pain which she had struggled with for years and was astonished at how this was considerably eased by some of the yoga asanas. Quite a few of the younger people there had come to the retreat as part of a de-addiction programme and Siobhan, as a former addict herself who had painfully become clean, soon became a sort of mother-confessor to them and started enjoying herself. It was great to see her slowly acclimatising to the unaccustomed exercise and healthy lifestyle, looking so much better and happier.

The food was astonishingly good too. Each vegetable dish was so full of flavour that one couldn't imagine needing either meat or alcohol to liven things up. Much less popular, but doubtless beneficial, was another branch of Ayurvedic medicine – panchakarma – various cleansing and purging systems whereby the body is purified by eliminating toxins. The oil massages (good) and daily dawn doses of medicated herbs (disgusting) were part of this. The worst bit though was when the serious purging began. We each had a morning set aside for this. Instead of breakfast we were given a concoction of herbs in ghee (clarified butter) and then spent the day within running distance of the bathroom. Each violent eruption had to be counted and noted down – the more the better. You could also choose to be made to vomit – an option I decided to forego.

We were left to our own devices in the afternoons and usually took little motorised carts down to the small town of Conoor or just wandered through the miles of green tea plantations surrounded by scented eucalyptus forests and blue mountains. At the end of the week, we were weighed. I was delighted – I had lost half a stone in the most pleasurable way imaginable, without ever feeling a hunger pang. And… it had given me the taste for yoga.

2

A Helping Hand

So, I had lost half a stone thanks to Ayurvedic massage and diet and you would think I would now be happy to plunge full time into yoga and to keep up the good work. But not a bit of it. Having lost a little weight, I now became dissatisfied with the weight I was still carrying, especially round my waist and stomach – an additional post-menopausal kick in the teeth that seems to affect most women.

And it was whilst doing yoga, ironically, that I decided to do something deeply un-yogic which will horrify most right-minded people, but since it is part of my story – here goes.

Things came to head when I was doing a shoulder stand – a difficult pose for beginners at the best of times. As my legs sailed up into the air, I noticed that not only was I struggling for breath, but that my stomach lurched forward to greet me in the most disagreeable way. This sagging lump of excess blubber, released from its normal stranglehold of support tights, was celebrating its freedom by slapping me in the face. It was far too slack to suck in, and as I looked around me at the other class members, hoping to spot a few similarly unre-strained bellies, all I could see were rows of washboard stomachs. It was a life-changing moment: the belly had to go and I knew that yoga wasn't going to do it fast enough.

That was why, three months later, as a birthday present to myself, I spent the morning lying on a hospital bed while a doctor took 2.3 litres of fat from my abdomen. The gift I was left with – a wonderfully flat stomach – made it all worthwhile.

Sound too good to be true? Well, let me tell you a story...

Once upon a time, there were a great many people who were dissatisfied with their appearance – usually, because they had eaten too much or drunk too much. Sometimes, the strong-willed ones managed to lose their lumps of unsightly fat by starving themselves or partaking in demonic exercise sessions, but others, in spite of really trying hard to exercise and diet, couldn't shift those fatty bits.

Others didn't even try. Then along came a U.S. doctor who invented an ultrasonic device called a Vaser which became his magic wand. He would wave this magic wand and dissolve the fatty bits and, hey presto, you had it sucked out and lived happily ever after. Now I don't make a habit of believing fairy stories like this, but after weeks of researching how to rid myself of my muffin top and discovering that, post menopause, nothing really works, I felt pretty desperate and willing to try anything.

But could cosmetic surgery really hold the answer?

Of course I had vaguely heard of tummy tucks, liposuction and such like, but I have never been interested in watching those grisly reality TV programmes, or even reading about it. I had always assumed I would never need it and, even if I did, would be too sensible to risk deformity or even death in the name of vanity.

However, after some research, I realised that things have moved on in the cosmetic surgery world and there were all kinds of new techniques for enhancing one's appearance which don't involve knives or general anaesthetics. My new obsession led me to YouTube, where I watched a film of a large lump of lard floating in a glass of water. A hand appeared with a sort of swizzle stick and after a moment the lard dissolved. I had to have that stick.

It turned out to be a promotional film for Vaser Liposuction, a patented technology which uses the gentle power of ultrasound to burst fat cells in just about any part of your body.

Apparently, this liquefied fat can then be easily and safely sucked out to produce instant results – or as the film's American presenter promises, 'a smokin' hot bod'!

At 58, the smokin' hot bod I could live without, but the thought of being able to wear jeans that didn't have flesh-coloured jelly spilling over the waistband was very appealing indeed. But could it really just be 'waved' away?

Vaser liposuction uses ultrasound technology and is

far less intrusive then traditional liposuction – it involves no cutting or blood – and is performed under local rather than general anaesthetic.

A small probe is inserted through a tiny incision, which transmits gentle ultrasound energy to break up fatty tissues. The liquefied fat is then removed through a suction process.

What distinguishes the Vaser is its ability to differentiate targeted fat from other important tissues (such as nerves, blood vessels and connective tissues, things you'd really rather keep) which are left intact. Even more appealing, the healing is relatively rapid and the effects are said to be permanent.

The technique received full accreditation in the U.S. in 2002, and is now in what practitioners call its third generation in terms of refinement. Curiously, it is still relatively unknown in this country.

When I told my friends and family, their initial reactions ranged from concern to extreme disapproval. 'That is just so unfair', exclaimed my daughter, overtly expressing what many dared not admit: jealousy or, as in my husband's case (he's a Scot), Calvinistic disapproval that I might get a good result in spite of not having worked to get it.

My friend Mary was more altruistic: horrified at the thought of the risks, she arranged for me to talk to a friend of hers, Charles McCollum, Professor of Surgery at Manchester University.

She thought he'd talk me out of it, but he is in fact the founder of one of best clinics in the country, one which carries out this procedure among many others, and he couldn't have been more enthusiastic. 'Vaser is a very effective, safe procedure,' he assured me. According to McCollum, Vaser is better than laser (the tool used to breakdown fat in a more common procedure known as SmartLipo).

Laser generates high local energies which vaporise tissues, and is almost impossible to control, risking small burns. With ultrasound, however, the frequency used to burst fat cells is very gentle, and it is suitable for almost everywhere on the body.

I started to shop around for suitable clinics and plumped for Dr Mike Comins at his Hans Place Practice in Knightsbridge. Dr Comins is president of the British Association of Cosmetic Doctors and one of the pioneers of the Vaser treatment in this country. He also gave Toyah Willcox the bum lift she raves about, so I felt in safe hands.

I prepared for my initial consultation by making myself watch videos online of beakers filling up with orange fat during Vaser procedures on U.S. patients, who reassuringly all had smiles on their faces and appeared to be in no discomfort at all – even though the pump action of the Vaser looked rather brutal. What was most impressive was the way they jumped up off the operating table at the end as though they'd just had a beauty treatment. One even went straight back to the office.

Dr Comins examined me and declared me a fit subject for the treatment. This is not a procedure for people who are very overweight and should not be regarded as the route to instant weight loss. 'It's a complement to a healthy lifestyle rather than a replacement for it', he explained.

I wanted to know what happens if you don't commit to a healthy lifestyle afterwards. Would you just put on weight in the same spot?

Dr Comins told me that if you experience weight gain after treatment, any fat would be proportionately distributed over your body. 'The treatment permanently gets rid of fat cells, but there will be a few left. However, you could put on as much as a stone without changing shape in the area.'

He assured me that the risks were few, before showing me a selection of before and after pictures of previous patients, some of whom had dropped four dress sizes.

On the morning of the procedure, I was surprised to find that I didn't feel too nervous. And, unlike with a general anaesthetic, I was allowed to eat breakfast. At the clinic, I gratefully accepted the valium I was offered while Dr Comin set to work marking out the areas to be treated on my body – around my stomach – which was swabbed with iodine. He then spent about 20 minutes administering what seemed like a vast amount of local anaesthetic.

Once I felt numb around the middle, he made three small incisions in my stomach and commenced treatment with the Vaser probe. I felt fine, but it looked awfully tiring for him – like very energetic ironing.

It felt like a scraping sensation inside, as if he was weeding my stomach with a trowel. It wasn't pleasant and I wanted it to end, but it wasn't painful due to the local anaesthetic.

We chatted intermittently as though all we were doing was waiting for a bus, but when the actual 'sculpting' got under way, I had to ask him to stop once or twice when I felt the odd twinge and tweak. It wasn't that it was agonisingly painful; it's like when you're having a filling under local anaesthetic and you occasionally feel the dentist touch a raw nerve.

After he finished with the ultrasound and the fat was liquefied, I watched with horrified interest as it was sucked out into a beaker. Not for the squeamish, but better out than in, I figured.

After an hour and a half, it was done. The nurse helped me into a support garment, which looked disconcertingly like bondage gear – a corset-like device, covered with hooks and eyes, which sucked me in from under the bust to below the knicker line.

I took a taxi home armed with painkillers and a course of antibiotics. Feeling pretty battered and tired, I didn't dare look at my stomach, as the incision wounds had been left open in order for the local anaesthetic to drain out.

The nurses had stuck large pads over the wounds, underneath the support garment, and I wasn't allowed to remove anything for the first 24 hours.

During that time, I slept as much as I could and,

once the discharge had stopped, I finally plucked up the courage to strip off the support garment and surveyed myself.

The wounds were healing well, but I was covered with purple and green bruises. However, nothing hurt acutely – I just felt a bit vulnerable and delicate.

By day three, I felt a lot better and took a bath (in spite of being told only to shower): the wounds had healed and I felt the need to escape from my corset, which itched horribly but was apparently necessary to keep on for at least two weeks for best results.

It wasn't until I found a tape measure that all that poking and prodding felt worthwhile: I'd lost three inches from my waist.

Obviously, there are risks to any invasive procedures, but I have to say that I was happy with the results. And I don't care what anyone says, it helps to have a boost like that to one's confidence before embarking on an exercise regime like yoga because it acts as such an incentive to maintain body shape and/or improve upon it.

A footnote to this story is that about a year later I choose to have my eyes lasered so that I didn't have to keep a pair of reading specs in every room. Again, the procedure was successful.

'Look at me', I said to my husband. 'I've been vasered, lasered…what next?'

'Tasered?' he suggested.

3

Stretching Yourself Healthy

'You are as young as your spine is flexible' is the motto for this chapter – something that makes perfect sense to me when you consider that it's what holds you together.

So, armed with some knowledge of yoga, I still needed to find more out about the potential benefits. I was especially interested in the anti-aging properties of regular practice.

As a journalist, I have a healthy scepticism about most things, but particularly about the kind of testimonials you find on the internet or elsewhere. In my research, I found hundreds of 'ordinary people' who attested that yoga had changed their lives (for the better, natch). But seeing is believing and I urge anyone interested to look at photographs and videos (on YouTube) of elderly 'ordinary' people in extraordinary yoga poses, as well as yoga masters like Tao Porchon-Lynch kicking her legs in the air at 93, and Iyengar himself (now in his nineties) who is still performing rigorous daily yoga practice. I was especially tickled by an account in Iyengar's biography, written by Kofi Busia, of him being introduced to the Queen Mother of Belgium in 1958 when she was already 85 years old: 'She wanted to learn to stand on her head and was not about to take No for an answer saying: 'if you can't teach me to stand on my head, you can leave''. The Queen was duly hoisted on to her head and survived the experience. Though sadly I can't find a photograph of the event.

But it was various contemporary accounts, by medical doctors and scientists, of the health and anti aging benefits of yoga that convinced me I was about to embark on a mission that could really roll back time. Dr Cynthia Bailey, a dermatologist in California, writes: 'The impact of adding yoga to my life is a marvel… I've only practised for two years and the anti aging impact is so profound that I know I've altered the course of my aging journey. My musculoskeletal problems were taking away more and more of my functionality. From what I have experienced, yoga has up-ed the odds that I'll age as a fit, functional, vital woman. I won't join the ranks of the frail elderly without a fight and yoga is one of the powerful puzzle pieces I've found to help me.'

Being a good doctor, she adds that she carried out medical literature research on the benefits of yoga and found that scientific study supported her own observations of yoga's benefits on her body and mind. Research shows that yoga: reduces low back pain; improves balance; straightens spinal kyphosis (excessive hunching up as people age); improves muscle strength and reverses muscle loss; improves symptoms of rheumatoid arthritis; improves menopausal symptoms; decreases anxiety and depression; improves control of type 2 diabetes and generally increases flexibility.

Sources for these commendations come from august institutions like The Buck Institute for Age Research and The Harvard Women's Health Watch. Her conclusion? 'I highly recommend three days a week of yoga for healthy aging'.

In 1990, headlines were made when a San Francisco cardiologist, Dr Dean Ornish, showed that heart disease can be reversed by combining yoga with changes in diet. To the astonishment of the medical establishment he proved that advanced heart patients could actually shrink the fatty plaque deposits that were progressively blocking their coronary arteries. Instead of taking the regular conventional route of drugs and surgery, Ornish's group used simple yoga exercises, meditation, and a strict low-cholesterol diet.

His study, 'The Lifestyle Heart Trial', with data published in the *Lancet* in 1990, is often cited because mainstream medicine had never before acknowledged that heart disease could actually be reversed once it had started. Not only did patients assigned to his regimen fare better than those who followed standard medical advice, they had narrower coronary arteries at the end of the trial than the start. After another study in 1998, in which 80 per cent of the 194 heart patients in the experimental group were able to avoid bypass or angioplasty by adhering to lifestyle changes, Ornish was quoted as saying that he was convinced that 'adherence to the yoga and meditation program was as strongly correlated with the changes in the amount of blockage as was the adherence to the diet.'

Ornish, founder and president of the non-profit Preventative Medicine Research Institute in Sausalito, California, has spent over 30 years conducting a series of scientific studies demonstrating that lifestyle can reverse heart disease. He was named by *Life* as one of the most 50 influential members of his generation, and acknowledges his debt to the yogi, Shri Swami Satchidananda, with whom he has studied yoga.

A consultant physician to President Clinton and author of five best-selling books, he is one of the scientists who has done the most to promote yoga as an acceptable part of modern American medicine. 'When I first began conducting research 23 years ago,' he says, 'we had to refer to yoga as 'stress management techniques'. The cardiologists said, 'we can't refer to a study that includes yoga – what are we going to tell patients, that we're referring them to a swami?' Since then yoga has achieved much greater acceptance within medical circles as well as in the general population.' Medicare is currently funding his Preventative Medicine Research Institute's research into the benefits of his yoga and diet regimen for elderly heart patients at hospitals nationwide.

Increasingly, yoga is being used by physiotherapists and sport therapists to treat patients with back injuries in particular. In Britain, the Yoga Biomedical Trust is researching yoga therapy for back pain. And in a different field, the MD Anderson Cancer Centre in Houston, Texas has recently received the largest yoga research grant to date – £2.8m – for a project researching the benefits of using yoga in treating breast cancer.

Deepak Chopra, the Indian medical doctor who was an established endocrinologist before shifting his focus to alternative medicine, points out one of the differences in approach between conventional medicine and alternative medicine in one of his books, which helps explain why Ornish's findings were considered so interesting: 'We all tend to see our bodies as 'frozen sculptures' – solid, fixed material objects – when, in truth, they are more like rivers, constantly changing flowing patterns of intelligence. If you pinch an inch around your waist, the fat you are squeezing between your fingers is not the same as it was last month. Your adipose tissue (fat cells) fill up with fat and empty out constantly so all of it is exchanged every three weeks.'

Chopra now runs his own medical centre with an emphasis on mind-body connections. A friend of Michael Jackson's for a number of years, he was widely quoted after Jackson's death from an overdose of a prescription drug as criticising 'the cult of drug-pushing doctors, with their co-dependent relationships with addicted celebrities'.

Another great source of inspiration and information is

The New Yoga for People over 50 by Suza Francina, a highly respected Iyengar yoga instructor since 1972 and a pioneer in the field of teaching yoga to 'seniors'. Yes, I had to gulp at that word too; surely I'm still an infant – I certainly behave like one at times as my family will attest.

Punctuated with photographs of elderly people doing the kind of things many young people can only dream of, like handstands and shoulder stands, Suza Francina's mantra is that you're never too old to do yoga. On the contrary, you're too old *not* to do yoga. 'No segment of our population can benefit more from yoga than people over 50. In fact, the older you are, the more you will benefit. Yoga goes against the grain by removing the stiffness and inertia from the body.' People of all ages, she says, generally start yoga to stretch the 'kinks' out of their body, to strengthen their bones and muscles, to improve their posture, to breathe better, to relax and improve their overall health and vitality. Older students who attend the class regularly for at least six months report that their increased strength and range of movement enables them to return to physical activities they thought they had lost for ever.

Throughout the book are truly inspiring photos, quotes and personal stories of teachers and students from all over the world, many in their 70s and older, who demonstrate that age is irrelevant when it comes to benefitting from yoga practice. Featured, for example, are Diana Clifton, a highly respected teacher in her mid-70s; Vanda Scaravelli, born in 1908, and author of *Awakening the Spine*; Indra Devi, who at 94, was still travelling the world, lecturing on the benefits of yoga and Frank White demonstrating an advanced balance pose at the age of 76. White, I should add, started yoga aged 66 when it was becoming increasingly difficult for him to get out of bed in the morning since he had severe degenerative osteoarthritis. When he started doing yoga regularly he lost 50 pounds, his blood pressure returned to normal without medication and his cholesterol dropped from 400 to 150.

OK, by now I'm almost convinced. I pause at this point to tell my husband (with whom I'm reunited) that not long ago there were photographs in the news of two of America's oldest sisters, Sarah and Elizabeth Delany, then ages 102 and 104 – one doing a shoulder stand, the other stretching in a yoga pose with one foot behind her head. 'Well, it's a message to us all', he says languidly, drawing on a large cigar.

But I find I can't stop reading about the miracle of yoga and its benefits (as opposed at this point to just getting on with it). Another remarkable book by a doctor presents itself: *Yoga as Medicine: the Yogic Prescription for Health & Healing* by Timothy McCall MD. This is known as the definitive book of yoga therapy and of course Iyengar pops up again at the beginning with a fitting epigraph: 'Words fail to convey the total value of yoga. It has to be experienced.' Yes, I know, I really do, but I've just got to read a bit more of this eye-popping stuff before I unroll my mat:

McCall, like so many others, came to yoga in middle age and found it 'incredibly challenging'. But, he says, 'my body has changed in ways I wouldn't have believed possible, as has my mental state'. Astonished by the changes yoga had wrought in his own body, he began investigating the use of yoga for people suffering from a variety of medical conditions. Echoing my own worries in this area, he found it difficult since there is no one place to acquire this knowledge.

'The yoga world is incredibly balkanized. There are dozens of competing traditions, many of which don't seem interested in sharing their discoveries with each other or the outside world. Complicating matters further, some of what I've heard from yoga teachers, or read in magazines, quite frankly defies modern understanding of anatomy and physiology, or is grounded in a metaphysics that can be off-putting or virtually incomprehensible. In addition, many yoga teachers with much to offer are shy about touting yoga's therapeutic potential – especially in writing – while others who in my estimation have far less substance, boldly claim their brand of yoga can cure any disease.'

Not to be deterred, he read widely, attended classes, workshops and conferences, reviewed the scientific literature and sought out some of the world's leading yoga teachers and therapists to find out what they were doing and what they found most helpful (you hear from many of these in this book). He also worked with his own teacher, Patricia Walden, using yoga to treat people with depression, breast cancer and Parkinson's disease.

Everything he saw convinced him, with his years of clinical medical experience, that yoga is an effective treatment for a variety of problems from heart disease to carpal tunnel syndrome.

'My experience tells me yoga works – in addition, of course, to the scientific evidence and what I've directly observed and heard from others. My suggestion is to suspend disbelief just long enough to try a few sessions of yoga and let your experience dictate whether to continue. If you find yoga brings you nothing, you won't have lost much. But if you find the experience as eye-opening as I have, you have a whole world to gain.'

'As someone who had been an MD for over twenty years, I can tell you that yoga is quite simply the most powerful system of overall health and well-being I have ever seen. Even if you are currently among what might be called the temporarily healthy, as preventative medicine, yoga is as close to one-stop shopping as you can find. This single comprehensive system can reduce stress, increase flexibility, improve balance, promote strength, heighten cardiovascular conditioning, lower blood pressure, reduce being overweight, strengthen bones, prevent injuries, lift mood, improve immune function, increase the oxygen supply to the tissues, heighten sexual functioning and fulfilment, foster psychological equanimity, and promote spiritual well-being... and, that's only a partial list.'

Throughout, McCall is keen to stress that yoga is not in competition with Western medicine, rather it complements it (a survey released in December 2008 by the

US National Center for Complementary and Alternative Medicine found that yoga was the sixth most commonly used alternative therapy in the United States during 2007). He is careful to emphasise that if you do suffer from such illnesses, you do not just wander into a random yoga class near you and join in. It is important to do the research first.

It is worth summarising his findings about the main benefits of yoga on different parts of the body and mind:

Improved flexibility: One of the most obvious benefits. Even though when you start, you probably will be unable to touch your toes, never mind do a backbend, if you stick with it, you'll notice you become looser and that familiar aches and pains will disappear. Your hamstrings will lengthen and this is important as tight hamstrings can lead to a flattening of the lumbar spine, which can cause backache. Also your hips will become more open. Tight hips can strain the knee joint due to improper alignment of the thigh and shinbones.

Strength: Yoga builds up strength and strong muscles protect you from conditions such as arthritis and back pain, and help prevent falls.

Joints: Joints are taken through their full range of motions in a yoga practice. This can help prevent degenerative arthritis by 'squeezing and soaking' areas of cartilage that normally aren't used.

Neglected cartilage eventually wears out like worn-out brake pads and needs fresh supplies of nutrients.

Spine: Spinal disks, the shock absorbers between the vertebrae, crave nutrients through movement. Yoga helps to keep them supple through backbends, forward bends and twists.

Bones: The weight bearing asanas in yoga – many of which require you to take your own weight – strengthen bones. Downward and Upward Facing Dog for example, strengthen the arm bones which are particularly vulnerable to osteoporotic fractures.

Blood: Yoga gets your blood flowing and gets more oxygen into your cells which function better as a result. Twisting poses are thought to wring out venous (de-oxygenated) blood from internal organs and allow oxygenated blood to flow in when the twist is released. Inverted poses such as headstand, handstand and shoulder stand encourage venous blood from the legs and pelvis to flow back to the heart where it can be pumped to the lungs to be freshly oxygenated. Yoga also boosts levels of haemoglobin and red blood cells which carry oxygen to the tissue. It thins the blood by making platelets less sticky and by cutting down clot-promoting proteins in the blood.

Lymphatic System: When you contract and stretch

muscles and move organs around, you increase the drainage of lymph which helps the lymphatic system fight infection, destroy cancerous cells and dispose of toxic waste.

Heart: Yoga is known to lower blood pressure and the risk of heart attack.

Weight: A regular practice burns calories.

Blood Sugar and Cholesterol: Yoga lowers blood sugar and bad cholesterol while boosting good cholesterol. It lowers blood sugar by lowering cortisol and adrenaline levels.

Breath: Yogis are taught to take fewer breaths of greater volume which is both calming and more efficient. A 1998 study published in the *Lancet* taught a yogic technique known as 'complete breathing' to people with lung problems due to congestive heart failure. After one month, their average respiratory rate decreased from 13.4 breaths per minute to 7.6.

Immune system: Likely that both asanas and pranayama (breathing techniques) improve immune function, but meditation has the strongest scientific support in this area (see later chapter).

Bowels: Yoga, like any physical exercise, can ease constipation and irritable bowel syndrome. The twisting poses are thought to be beneficial in getting waste to move through the system.

Pain Control: Yoga can ease pain, especially in people with arthritis, back pain, fibromyalgia, carpal tunnel syndrome, and other chronic conditions.

And that's just your body, I haven't even touched on what it can do for your mind. Both doctors and patients have claimed that it combats stress, worry, depression, and insomnia for starters. It also promotes relaxation, peace and a quiet mind. Others go further and claim that it boosts self-esteem and confidence too.

As a seasoned unbeliever, I was completely worn down by this book. I wanted to take the next plane out to Boston and bring McCall home with me. Once I had read the book through at one sitting on my kindle, I ordered a hard copy for good measure and told everyone I met to do the same. McCall gets you on side straight away by confessing his own initial scepticism. Then, with commendable academic restraint, he takes you through his own experiences and research, and cites such a wealth of evidence and case-studies to support his theories that you would have to be exceptionally blinkered not to keep an open mind. I urge people disposed to scoff, like me, or even just the intellectually curious to read just the first couple of chapters before switching off the telly, leaping off the sofa and running down the road to find a yoga class. I know it's time I did…

4

The Yoga File

I have the kind of anal personality which dictates that I won't do anything until I've researched it, approved it, bought the uniform and told everybody what I'm about to do. As far as yoga was concerned, I'd had one unsatisfactory experience and whilst I was intrigued by all the purported benefits, I certainly wasn't going to try it again until I knew exactly what the practice itself was all about.

Yoga is a system of physical, mental and spiritual development: it is not a religion or creed, and it can be practised by any one of any age and by either sex. According to the British Wheel of Yoga, the yogis succeeded in discovering how the body works and how they could consciously direct their energies towards sustaining health, vigour and the prolongation of their life span. Each asana (posture) is designed to have a specific, beneficial effect upon the functioning of the body. Sometimes it will be to regain or maintain the suppleness of muscles or joints, or it may be concerned with enriching the blood supply to certain glands. Other postures may, combined with certain breathing techniques, massage the internal organs. However, the ultimate aim of yoga is to attain 'self-realisation'.

Yoga is said to have originated in the Indus Valley Civilization at least 3000 years ago in what is now Pakistan and northwest India where archaeologists unearthed statuettes of men seated in what appears to be lotus position.

The word 'yoga' is derived from a Sanskrit word 'yui' meaning to bind, to unite or to yoke. It appears in the oldest Sanskrit text, the Rig Veda, only in this primary sense of 'yoking' (horses to chariots or animals to ploughs). But sometime in the middle of the first millennium BC in the Sanskrit philosophical texts known as the Upanishads, the word yoga designates the joining or yoking of body and mind – a spiritual praxis of meditation and breath control. It was also taken to be the union of man's will with that of God. It is in the Upanishads that yoga begins to take a more definable shape.

When I started researching yoga, and before I started to practise it in earnest, the God thing which crops up everywhere in the classic texts was troubling to me, as it is to many others in the West who just want to swing into action with the postures and to hell with all the mumbo jumbo. But of course one must respect the origins of yoga and the beliefs of those who practised it thousands of years ago. Indeed, Iyengar reminds his infidel Western readers in his introduction to *Light on Yoga* that in ancient times all the achievements of men 'even in the Western world' such as

music, art, architecture, medicine and philosophy –
even wars – were always offered up in the service of
God. That was the whole point. He adds, quite rightly,
that it is only recently in India that these arts and sci-
ences 'have begun to be emancipated from the Divine
– but with due respect... we in India continue to value
the purity of purpose, the humility of discipline and
the selflessness that are the legacy of our long bondage
to God.'

The Bhagavad-Gita, the seminal Hindu scripture
which is considered a kind of manual for mankind (and
has been venerated by the likes of Einstein, Jung,
Huxley and Hesse, as well as being Gandhi's great inspi
ration), goes further saying that yoga destroys all pain
and sorrow through moderation in all things and skilful
living. Indeed, even secular explanations of yoga will
not just emphasise the physical aspects of it, but also
the importance of attaining mental balance – the
perfect harmony between body and mind through
which we achieve self-realisation.

This made perfect sense to me and I realised that
one can practise yoga with or without God at the fore-
front of one's mind. What to some may be called
'God', to me, might be better termed 'peace' or 'a sense
of well-being'.

Indeed, the idea of focusing on both the body and
the mind, and the interaction between the two, as outlined in the Yoga Sutras (a corpus of work defining the
'sutras' or aphorisms on the philosophy and practice of
yoga) compiled in the years between 300 BC and 300

AD by the sage Patanjali, was extraordinarily perceptive and ahead of its time. Nowadays, we take for granted that the body and mind interact when physical acts affect brain chemistry. Brain scanners now show us that different parts of the brain light up when a physical action occurs. But back then, it must have been entirely intuitive and/or the result of experimentation and observation. Yoga has always assumed that body and mind were a single integrated entity – that is if you achieve physical harmony, then mental harmony follows. In the final chapter of the Yoga Sutras, the Samadhi Pada, Patanjali discusses the disorders which are the root cause of suffering. Physical ailments, he insists, create emotional upheaval. The task of yoga is to tackle both.

The basic tenets of yoga are described by Patanjali in the form of 'eight limbs' or steps (the basis of Ashtanga yoga). Each step must be understood and followed to attain the ultimate goal – the emancipation of the self. Anyone who has ever had to join Alcoholics Anonymous or any group for addiction will recognise this kind of step system. In yoga, briefly, these are:

1. Yama: (Moral Codes): five universal moral commandments of non violence, truthfulness, freedom from greed, chastity, freedom from desire.
2. Niyama: (Self purification and study): five personal disciplines of cleanliness, contentment, austerity, study of one's own self, devotion to God.

3. Asana: practice of the yoga postures
4. Pranayama: practice of breathing control
5. Pratyahara: sensory transcendence
6. Dharana: Concentration
7. Dhyana: Meditation
8 Samadhi: (Contemplation): Liberation of Self
– trance-like state of Bliss (the final goal)

From this, you can see that Asana, the third limb of yoga (practising the physical postures) is but one of the branches of yoga, keeping the body healthy and strong and in harmony with nature. But, at first, this was the only one that even remotely interested me in my quest for youth and good health. I'm afraid no-one could accuse me of being naturally yogic: looking at all those commandments. I could say, hand on heart, that I was pretty clean and didn't go in for much violence, but my self discipline was pretty shaky and my devotion to God non-existent. As for meditation, I just knew I was far too twitchy and self-absorbed to do that. And Bliss? Well, that was obviously a good night's sleep as far as I was concerned.

In the middle ages, people known as Yogis were more often than not ascetics who, instead of celebrating their bodies, cultivated 'the aversion to one's own body' in punishing ways by subjecting themselves to extremes of heat and cold, fasting, and other forms of physical mortification such as standing on one leg for days at a time (something you can still see in India and is described by Gregory David in *Shantaram*, his dazzling largely autobiographical novel about his life in Bombay). They were reviled as lunatics and also were seen to pose a sexual threat, because of an ancient Hindu belief in their erotic powers. Their reputation was sullied further later on by the overlap between yoga and Tantric techniques (think Sting and Trudie). By this time, most educated Hindus scorned postural yoga, though there was still respect for yoga as a spiritual discipline. Indeed, well-born Bengalis apparently considered exercise in general to be very lower-class, an attitude that gave rise to Noel Coward's line: 'In Bengal, to move at all is seldom, if ever, done.'

Interestingly, Mark Singleton's groundbreaking scholarly book, *Yoga Body: The origins of modern posture practice*, calls into question many commonly held beliefs that the roots of modern yoga lie in ancient India and their Vedic texts. His surprising thesis is that yoga as it is popularly practised today owes a greater debt to modern Indian nationalism (when militant Yogis engaged in exercise regimes to make them tough enough to oppose the British under the Raj), the British obsession with bodybuilding and the early 20th century women's gymnastic movements of Europe and America, than it does to any ancient Indian yoga tradition. There is of course evidence for yoga in the ancient Indian texts but it is not the source of what most people regard as yoga today.

Singleton argues that in the 20th century a transnational Anglophone yoga arose, compounded by the culture of British bodybuilding, American Christian

Science, Swedish gymnastics and, most of all, by the
YMCA, an institution which made physical culture
socially and morally acceptable. YMCA leaders in India
had made yoga postures part of the physical programme in service of Christian goals, and the British
passion for physical culture rescued physical yoga from
the opprobrium into which it had fallen. This new yoga
took the European techniques and couched them in the
Vedantic language of the Upanishads. This form of
yoga then travelled back to England. Even Queen
Victoria had eighteen audiences with Shivapuri Baba,
the first modern yoga guru to transplant the wisdom of
India to the west. It is not known, however, if she ever
stood on her head.

The most influential yogi of them all though, who
could be said to be the real founder of modern yoga
practice, was T. Krishnamacharya, who between 1930
and 1950 developed a novel sequence of movements,
partially derived from the royal gymnastic tradition in
Mysore. He was the teacher of both B.K.S. Iyengar and
K. Pattabhi Jois (who popularised Ashtanga yoga), and
believed 'Yoga to be India's greatest gift to the world'.
Krishnamacharya believed that every person is
'absolutely unique' and he felt that the most important
part of teaching yoga was that the student must be
'taught according to his or her individual capacity at any
given time. This means that the path of yoga will mean
different things for different people and each person
must be taught in a manner that they understand
clearly.'

Krishnamacharya was not only a yoga instructor, he was also considered a physician of Ayurvedic medicine and possessed enormous knowledge of nutrition, herbal medicine, the use of oils, and other remedies and he incorporated physical healing into his yoga teaching. Once a person began seeing Krishnamacharya, he would work with him or her on a number of levels including adjusting their diet, creating herbal medicines, and setting up a series of yoga postures that would be most beneficial.

And here's the bit I find particularly impressive: Krishnamacharya was known to be able to voluntarily stop his visible heart beat/ pulse for over two minutes, probably by drastically reducing venous return to the heart.

The British, thanks to their colonial interests, have always had an interest in Eastern religions and practices. In the late 19th century, Swami Vivekananda (1863-1902) increased awareness in the UK of the Vedantic texts by giving lectures in 'practical Vedanta' in London, and Annie Besant, an early feminist and reformer, and one time president of the Theosophical Society, who had moved to India, even published *An Introduction to Yoga* in 1908. Another formidable lady, Mary Bagot Stack (1883-1935) founded the Women's League of health and beauty in London in 1930 and her physical fitness programme incorporated yoga exercises learned while living in India with her soldier husband.

In the 1940s Desmond Dunne opened a School of

Yogism in London and Sir Paul Dukes, a famous British secret agent and master spy in Russia (a role for which he was knighted) as well as one time British ambassador to India, became the first proper western teacher of yoga in London. He also did much to popularise it in the rest of the UK by presenting a four part series of yoga demonstrations on BBC television in 1950 and by publishing several influential books on yoga.

In fact, my friend Sarah's Aunt Mary, a wonderful woman in her 90s when I met her, told me of her friendship with Paul Dukes and what an influence his books and his teachings had on her. 'It transformed my life,' she said. And she was still practising yoga very late in her life and looking every inch a grand ambassador for the yogic lifestyle until her death in 2011.

Like so many other things, yoga teaching really took off in the 1960s in the UK, when everything Indian from music and fashion to philosophy and religion became the ultimate in cool. In 1960 B.K.S. Iyengar gave public lectures and demonstrations in Highgate, London while staying there to teach yoga to Yehudi Menuhin. In 1961 Wilfred Clark (one of the founders of the British Wheel of Yoga) gave his first lectures on yoga to the Workers' Educational Association in Birmingham, while Maharishi Mahesh Yogi held a public meeting in the Royal Albert Hall on Transcendental Meditation.

George Harrison took sitar lessons from Ravi Shankar; the Wheel of Yoga held its first public rally in Birmingham; the Beatles declared their faith in meditation and reincarnation on the David Frost show on national television; Swami Prabhupada (founder of Krishnaism) shared the stage with The Grateful Dead; Iyengar yoga was approved in the ILEA curriculum; Terence Stamp turned his back on celebrity and boarded a plane for India; orange-clad people chanted 'Hari Krishna' on Oxford Street and my generation floated around in Indian cheesecloth shirts and declared ourselves to be Buddhists (I thought it just meant being kind to animals, especially cows).

In America, the popularisation of yoga followed a similar timeline. In 1893, Swami Vivekananda got a 3 minute standing ovation from an audience of 4000 people when he addressed the World's Parliament of Religions in Chicago on the religious and philosophical values of India – a speech which attracted many students to yoga and Vedanta. According to his biographer, Ann Louise Bardach, he had 'held the conference's attendees spellbound in a series of show stopping improvised talks. He had simplified Vedanta thought to a few teachings that were irresistible to Westerners, foremost being that 'all souls are potentially divine'. His prescription for life was simple, and perfectly American: 'Work and Worship'.

Vivekananda's followers included Leo Tolstoy, William James, Aldous Huxley, Christopher Isherwood, Henry Miller and J.D. Salinger. As far as yoga was concerned, his message was simple and meant just one thing – 'realising God'. A message that would be largely incomprehensible to yogis today.

In 1919, Yogendra Mastamani taught what might be called the first regular hatha yoga classes in upstate New York and wrote popular books on yoga asana for better health in English. The following year Paramahansa Yogananda founded the Self-Realization fellowship in California and wrote *Autobiography of a Yogi* which has sold millions of copies worldwide.

Not all yogis were entirely above board however, and America's largely puritanical reaction to yoga asanas and the kind of people who practised them in the 1920s was only heightened by an enterprising charlatan calling himself Pierre Bernard (born Perry Baker in Iowa) or the 'The Great Oom' who jumped on the yoga bandwagon and set up an exclusive members-only club called The Tantrik Order which was rumoured to be more of a love cult than anything else. The rich and famous flocked to his Manhattan school and it wasn't long before he was charged with holding a young girl hostage – enraptured by his 'psychic power'. The charges were dropped but the scandal drove Bernard to upstate NY where he and his followers settled in Nyack and the likes of the Vanderbilts and other trust fund families patronised him, helping to fund his increasingly fabulous lifestyle.

Later, Indra Devi, the sari-clad Swedish-Russian star of 1940s Bombay cinema and one of the cast of colourful eccentrics who brought yoga to America, only seems to have attracted the A list – this time in Hollywood. Greta Garbo, Gloria Swanson and Jennifer Jones were amongst those who tried yoga in Devi's studios. Marilyn Monroe claimed that yoga improved her legs.

By the 1950s, a book called *Sport and Yoga* by a prominent teacher Selvarajan Yesudian meant that a lot of athletes began incorporating yoga into their workouts. In the 1960s Richard Hittleman, a prolific author on yoga practice, brought Hatha Yoga to mainstream television.

Since then, yoga has become increasingly popular – less so perhaps in the 1980s when it was eclipsed by the trend for more aggressive workouts like aerobics – but it made a comeback in the 1990s when Ashtanga yoga and Bikram yoga – both strenuous workouts, the latter practised in a hot room – gained explosive popularity.

At the time of writing, it is estimated that almost 20 million Americans practise some kind of yoga – three times as many as practise Judaism for example.

5

Striking a Pose: Asanas

I don't mean to boast (un-yogic as well as unattractive) but I was the school champion at walking on my hands. I could also (as indeed many of us could) stand for ages on my head, do a backbend from standing and do the splits. It comes as an unpleasant surprise, therefore, when I finally find the right yoga class and teacher some four years after my first foray into yoga, to find that I can't even touch my toes. And it's agony to sit cross-legged, let alone in lotus. I seem to have forgotten that half a century has gone by since then, not to mention the children I have delivered and the tons of unwholesome things I have ingested.

I think it's the shock of realising that I have neglected my body since I was ten that spurs me on initially. It is frustrating and humiliating not to be able to do what other people in my class (some years older than me) are doing and it occurs to me that if I don't look out, I will become one of those old people who shuffle along in pain, bent double and wondering where it all went wrong.

So I persist and this is what happens. The teacher is patient and gentle; the other people in the class do not mock, or even notice, how stiff I am. Over the course of a few weeks, I improve quite dramatically. My 'muscle memory' has returned: my body can apparently recall what it's supposed to be able to do and points in the right direction. I learn that I can breathe into the poses – a really important revelation – and my confidence begins to build up. I find I like doing yoga – I *love* it in fact, now that I'm getting better. I even get quite cocky and look around the class to see if my ankles are closer to the ground in downward dog than anyone else's. I am reprimanded for this ('It's not a competition, Carla!')

What's more, it feels so good to be stretched out. My back, particularly, is grateful. All my aches and twinges have gone. My spine has evidently been crying out for some exercise. I can hardly wait to lie on my back and swing my legs over to each side (Jathara Parivatanasana). I like the sound of the Sanskrit names of the poses and gradually learn to recognise them. I am charmed by the fact that many of them take their names from animals and insects, and that some of them are things that children all over the world do naturally in parks in playgrounds (or they used to) like handstands and headstands and the Wheel without knowing they are doing yoga. I feel I have found a form of exercise that I don't dread – that I look forward to. I feel I have come home.

Important things I learn:

How to relax
How to stretch every muscle
How to take my own body weight on my hands
How to balance
How to breathe properly through my nose
How to sit up and stand up straight

I realise that this is the most anti-ageing thing I have ever done. Forget the botox, the vaser, the laser, the facials and the whole cosmetic approach – that's fine too, but only as an add-on. Your body needs to be nourished – every muscle, every gland, every organ needs to work in order to fulfil its purpose. And when your body works, your mind follows. It's a revelation!

True to form, I buy lots of yoga books and find out as much as I can about Hatha yoga – the physical side of yoga, the third limb in which the student gains mastery over his body through practising the asanas and pranayama. Once the body is under control, then the student can concentrate on gaining control over the mind through meditation. Once they have done that too, they are ready to proceed along the eightfold path of Raja yoga, though most of us are quite content to stay with the body and breath since the physical body, the outermost aspect of the personality, is a practical starting point.

Estimates of the number of asanas (asana is the Sanskrit word for seat) vary – some say 600, some say thousands. According to Swami Satyananda Saraswati, the author of the book yoga teachers swear by (*Asana*

Pranayama Mudra Bandha), the yogic scriptures say there were originally 8,400,000 asanas, which represent the 8,400,000 incarnations every individual must pass through before attaining liberation from the cycle of birth and death. These asanas represented a progressive evolution from the simplest form of life to the most complex – a fully realised human being.

Dharma Mittra, the well known New York yogi, famously compiled a *Master Yoga Chart* of 908 Postures in 1984 after having meticulously photographed himself in 1300 poses. But there are maybe 50-100 'core' asanas which you come across in most classes. Many of them have animal names such as Camel, Dog, Rabbit, Crow, Cobra and Fish supposedly based on yogis observing such animals in the wild.

The asanas are based on a sound knowledge of human anatomy and physiology. Yogis knew that by placing the body in certain positions, they would stimulate specific nerves, organs and glands. For example, the shoulder stand posture causes blood to be directed by gravity to the thyroid gland, and the tucking in of the chin causes the gland to be squeezed. These two actions have a profound beneficial effect on the thyroid gland.

One of the main aims of asanas is to release mental tensions by dealing with them on the physical level – through the body to the mind. Muscular knots can occur anywhere in the body. We are familiar with tension carried in the form of knots in the shoulders and back but all kinds of conditions like neuralgia in the face and asthma are physical manifestations of stress. The asanas can help ease these tensions and release dormant energy. Regular practise therefore keeps the body and mind in optimum condition and promotes health and increased vitality and confidence. Broadly, the asanas fall into the following categories: sitting, standing, forward bends, back bends, twists, inversions, balances and reclining. A balanced practice would include a few of each, though the sequence in which they are performed needs to be thought out carefully for maximum benefit. Each type of yoga pose has its own purpose and benefits.

Sitting: According to Iyengar, all sitting poses bring elasticity to the hips, knees, ankles and muscles of the groin. They include: Rod or Staff (Dandasana); Hero (Virasana) and Cobbler (Baddha Konasana).

Standing: These strengthen the leg muscles, spine and joints. They are cardio-vascular and bring heat up into the body. They include: Mountain (Tadasana); Triangle (Trikonasana) and Warriors I and II (Virabhadrasana I and II). Some of them require balancing on one leg such as Tree (Viriksasana); Half Moon (Ardha Chandrasana) and Eagle (Garudasana).

Forward Bends: These are performed both sitting and standing involving bending the head towards the feat compressing the abdomen and toning the abdominal muscles. According to Iyengar, these can reduce stress and regulate blood pressure. They stretch the back and hamstring muscles and include: Standing Forward Bend (Uttanasana): Seated Forward Bend (Paschimottanasana) and Seated Wide Leg Forward Bend (Upavistha Konasana).

Twists: These can be performed whilst sitting, standing or lying down and involve twisting at the abdomen. All twisting poses massage and detoxify the internal organs. Twisting to the right compresses the large intestine, the liver and the right kidney. Twisting to the left compresses the pancreas, spleen and left kidney. All are flushed with fresh, oxygenated blood and perform better as a result. Twists are excellent for stimulating the endocrine system and wringing out the spine forcing out all the stale blood between the vertebrae. When the twist is released, the vacuum is refilled with fresh, oxygenated blood. They include: Seated Spinal Twist (Marichyasana); Lying Twist (Jathara Parivartanasana) and Simple Twist (Bharadvajasana).

Inversions: Any yoga position where the heart is placed above the head. These gravity-defying poses are amongst the most beneficial of all, enhancing both your body and mind. All blood is drained from extremities and again replaced by freshly oxygenated blood. The scalp and the brain are flushed with blood which can promote hair growth. But best of all, from my point of view, inversions like standing on your head help remove or fill out the small creases round the eyes and mouth which form due to lack of blood. This is a natural face lift, girls! Inversions also help the process of reversing collapsing organs. Human beings were designed to walk on all fours and their internal organs to stay in the same place. When we staggered to our feet, the force of gravity pulled everything downwards. We could get away with this if our lives were as physical as they once were, but nowadays almost everybody leads an unhealthily sedentary life which turns us into saggy sacks.

Inversions include: Downward Facing Dog (Adho Mukha Svanasana); Headstand (Sirshasana) and Shoulder Stand (Sarvangasana). The headstand is known as the King of Asanas because it stimulates the pituitary and pineal glands and allows the blood to flow freely to the brain feeding the brain cells with fresh oxygen. They also require strength and balance and, it is often said, if you only do one pose a day, this is the one to practise. Shoulder stand too, which is a little less demanding, has many of the same effects – massaging the thyroid and parathyroid glands, reversing gravity which helps drain and remove stagnant blood from extremities, and stimulating the immune system.

Yoga Journal reports that even the most basic of inverted postures (poses in which the heart is higher than the head) Legs up the Wall pose, and certainly the more difficult inverted postures, will help restore focus, improve sleep, relieve stress and depression and improve lymphatic drainage. Don't forget that Downward Dog is also an inverted pose and can be done using a chair or blocks until you gain flexibility, provides a great overall stretch, especially for the hamstrings, and the all-important rush of blood to the head.

Other important postures work on the glands. Somebody whose endocrine system is not working properly may suffer depression, be sluggish and obese. Again, the asanas work on the glands by increasing the blood supply to them. In a typical yoga practice, you will work on your pituitary gland (inverted postures), your thyroid gland (shoulder stands) as well as your pancreas, adrenal glands.

Backbends: Yoga positions where the spine is compressed and the front part of the body is open. They energise the body and stimulate the nervous system. Iyengar also recommends them for depression. People who are very introverted may benefit from these. They include: Cobra (Bhujangasana); Upward-Facing Dog (Urdhva Mukha Svanasana) and Bow (Dhanurasana).

Balances: Balance is crucial as we age. Everyone knows that when we start to fall over without imbibing alcohol, the end is probably round the corner. Balancing postures balance both sides of the brain – the right creative side and the left analytical side. They do wonders for co-ordination too. Standing balances like Mountain (Tadasana) and Tree (Viriksasana) promote good posture, help realign and balance the body, strengthen the leg muscles and calm the mind.

Sitting balances like Boat (Ardha Navasana) tone the abdominal organs, strengthen back muscles, tone kidneys and help achieve that nirvana of a trim waist.

Reclining Asanas: These are resting and restorative poses, performed lying down for longer periods of time. They include: Reclining Bound Angle Pose (Supta Baddha Konasana); Reclining Hero Pose (Supta Virasana) and Corpse (Savasana). Personally, by the time we reach Savasana at the end of a yoga class, I feel ten times more relaxed than I ever do in bed at night. Perhaps deep relaxation is only really possible after a physical workout.

But the asanas differ from mere physical exercise where muscle bulk is built up without regard for flexibility and only certain parts of the body are targeted. Asanas done in a certain sequence encompass the whole body – and each posture has a counter posture ensuring balance. Postures are done so that they put the body through a whole range of movements. More importantly, asanas must be approached with concentration and awareness – they are intended to benefit the mind as much as the body. Breath control is an integral part of the practice.

Some teachers will tell you that each posture should be approached as though you were doing it for the first time – it's not like doing 100 press-ups. Nothing should be rushed or forced. You are harnessing your body to your mind and this is what makes yoga unique. It also makes it a suitable form of exercise for everybody from children to pensioners. Restorative yoga which many doctors in the UK, and especially in the U.S., are starting to recommend is suitable for people recovering from serious operations as well as elderly and disabled people.

The benefits I have touched on before and they are legion, both for body and mind. For the body, obvious benefits are stamina, flexibility, toning, and circulation. Less obvious ones are that asanas work on the internal organs and the all-important endocrine system, regulating metabolism and improving the digestive and elimination process. Mentally, yoga calms and disciplines the mind, improving concentration, counteracting stress and giving control over unwanted emotion such as anger.

Particular attention in yoga asanas is given to the spine because, as we have already learnt, you are as old as your spine is flexible. The health of the spine is vital of course, housing as it does the spinal cord which carries instructions from the brain to the rest of the body and balancing your enormously heavy (20lb) head on top of it. Many asanas work on the spine by bending it forward, backward and through twisting movements. These ensure that the spinal nerves get a good supply of blood and that there are no blockages which cause back pain.

Finally, don't let's forget the brain. Thanks, once again, to brain imaging, we now know that many of the asanas, combined with proper breathing, contribute to a release of several essential chemicals or hormones in the body, which greatly enhances health. Inverted poses are amongst the most beneficial.

Among these chemical releases are: increased beta activity in the brain (characteristic of a strongly stimulated and engaged brain); increased release of feel good endorphin chemicals reducing stress and increasing a sense of well-being and happiness; increased gamma-aminobutyric acid (GABA) levels (decreasing risk of anxiety and depression since inadequate amounts of GABA are associated with a high risk of depression); the regulation of the level of dopamine in the brain (dopamine is a neuro-transmitter and many disorders, including Parkinson's disease, are associated dopamine deficiency).

And it does seem to be true. I always put down my good spirits after a yoga workout to that inglorious feeling of appalling smugness at having actually got off my arse and done some exercise, but if all the recent yoga and the brain studies are correct, I am actually wallowing in beta waves and endorphins.

The GABA studies are of especial interest to scientists. The *Daily Telegraph's* science correspondent reported that researchers found that three sessions of yoga a week can help fight off depression as it boosts levels of a chemical in the brain which is essential for a sound and relaxed mind.

Scientists found that the levels of the amino acid GABA are much higher in those that practise yoga than those who do the equivalent of a similarly strenuous exercise such as walking.

Favourite poses:

Back to asanas. I've been putting it off, but THE pose, the one everyone thinks of when they think of yoga is of course the meditative Lotus pose (Padmasana) in which the feet are placed, sole upwards, on the opposing thighs. And sooner or later any serious student of yoga is going to have to confront the idea of getting into this pose.

Carvings in India dating from around 3000 BC show figures sitting in lotus pose and it has its place in Hindu and Buddhist contemplative traditions. Famous depictions of the lotus position include Shiva, the meditative ascetic god of Hinduism, and Siddhartha Gautama, the founder of Buddhism.

The lotus is a symbol of purity, and the position is said to resemble a lotus. It is of course the ultimate hip opener and, for most of us, incredibly difficult to do. It helps to sit on the edge of a cushion (zafu) or mat (zabuton) in order to get the knees to make contact with the ground. When you can do it, it allows the body to be held completely steady for long periods of time which is conducive to meditation, the slowing of the breath and the decrease of muscular tension.

I am easily the worst in the class. My knees are nowhere near the floor, my feet obstinately refuse to turn over so that the soles are facing the ceiling, my ankles actually creak and my overriding emotion, far from meditative bliss, is rage. My teacher says it was her worst one too when she was learning, and that when she had exhausted her complaints to her teacher (my legs are too short, my thighs are too fat, my ankles hurt etc) she was left with just having to practise it every day. And it did the trick… eventually.

Another challenge in yoga is that you should practise at home as often as you can. Trying to put together your own practice is best discussed with a yoga teacher. Not only should you include poses from each of the categories, but also you should know what the counter-poses are and what your limitations are too. It is very tempting just to do the poses you are good at but obviously you wouldn't progress much if you did. On the other hand, everyone has their favourite poses and sometimes they are the ones that are most beneficial for you rather than the ones you can't do. It's important to listen to your body in that respect.

Finally, there seems to be some agreement in yoga blogs, magazines and chat forums over which poses are the best for women, and which for men.

For Women:

Child's pose (Balasana)
Downward Facing Dog (Adho Mukha Svanasana)
Plank (Chaturanga Dandasana)
Chair/Fierce pose (Utkatasana)
Warrior II (Virabhadrasana II)
Tree (Viriksasana)
Squat/Garland (Malasana)
Boat (Ardha Navasana)

Bridge (Setu Bandha)

For Men:

Wide-leg Forward Bend (Prasarita
Padottanasana)
Downward Facing Dog (Adho Mukha
Svanasana)
Chair (Utkatasana)
Crescent Lunge (Anjaneyasana)
Warrior I (Virabhadrasana I)
Bridge (Setu Bandha)
Bow (Dhanurasana)
Boat (Paripurna Navasana)
Hero (Virasana)
Reclining Big Toe (Supta Padangusthasana)

A straw poll among my yoga class which I thought
would produce pretty uniform results as to which yoga
poses they all preferred/thought were especially beneficial was surprising. There weren't any obvious
favourites – everyone had their own special ten best
poses.

My own, for what it's worth are:

Downward Dog
Triangle
Forward Bends (Standing, Wide Leg and Seated)
Pigeon

Handstand
Headstand
Locust
Crow
Shoulder Stand
Lying Twist
Camel

And, yes – Savasana (corpse pose) obviously. Probably the most relaxing part of any day – including the night.

6

When Yoga Hurts

My hamstring popped the other day, and boy did it hurt. We were in a partnered pose, legs wide apart, my feet propped against his ankles. As he lay backwards bringing me forward by the arms into a forward bend, we went down too fast and, shackled in this way, I couldn't monitor my movement. 'That could take a year to heal properly', said someone gloomily after the class.

As yoga has become popular, inevitably yoga injuries are on the increase and there are always people longing to tell you that their friend got a slipped disc or injured her rotator cuff doing yoga. It's talked about precisely because it's unexpected. Runners and bicyclists are fully aware that their knees are vulnerable; tennis players expect painful elbows and footballers never stop having leg injuries. But when yoga is prescribed by doctors for injured athletes, cancer and heart patients as an ancient healing discipline, one doesn't expect to hear that it's done more harm than good. And the fact that yoga is known to be good for you and heal injuries means that some people have such faith in it that they think a yoga teacher or yoga practice cannot possibly hurt them.

Reports both in the UK and the US highlight the surge in yoga-related injuries in recent years, but given the number of yoga practitioners, this isn't so surprising. Any form of physical exercise carries risks and hatha yoga is no exception, especially for people who push themselves too far, or are adjusted too aggressively by an inexperienced teacher.

Common injuries include overstretched neck, knees, spine, legs and wrists. Back injuries are frequent. Positions like upward dog and cobra in which the back is bent in one direction can aggravate the spine, as can the poses which elongate the back like seated forward bend which can wreak havoc on discs (I have heard more about slipped discs than any other injury just through chatting to other yogis). Rotator cuffs and wrists can take a hammering during plank poses and Chaturangas (like push-ups), while knees are susceptible to the lotus pose, hero's pose and the warrior positions.

The headstand is also an offender. If it is not done properly, or you attempt it before you are ready to do it and used to inversions, it can roil your back, neck, shoulders and wrists. Generally, inversions like the headstand and the shoulder stand should be avoided if you have cardiovascular problems, hypertension, diabetes or glaucoma. The Lotus position is another potentially dangerous pose. Without adequate hip-joint flexibility you could tear a meniscus or stretch or tear one of the knee ligaments.

In people over forty, the most common posture to

cause injuries is the shoulder stand, according to Larry Payne, a yoga teacher, therapist and co-author of *Yoga Rx*. Full shoulder stand can be dangerous for anyone carrying excess weight, as their neck will be very vulnerable to bone spurs, disc injuries, or worse.

Often, though, it's the very flexible people, or the hyper-flexible (those whose arms look like boomerangs when they stretch out) who are prone to injury as they can get pushed into poses too deeply.

One of the main reasons people injure themselves is because they come into class with an underlying condition and fail to tell the teacher. It is important to know your own condition before entering the class. One teacher told me how extraordinary it is that people who, for example, know they have carpal tunnel syndrome will still want to perform poses which put excess weight on the wrists: 'They think that because they are doing yoga, they are somehow protected.'

Then there are the freak accidents. I read of a woman doing the crow pose who fell on her face and broke her nose (only surprise is that this doesn't happen more often); the man who twisted his head to look at his teacher while in headstand and suffered long-lasting neck injury; the woman whose hip replacement was dislodged during a class, and, worse of all, a woman who hyper extended her neck in fish pose and suffered a stroke. It was found she had torn her left carotid, one of the two arteries located in the front of the neck that supply the head with blood, causing a clot which travelled to her brain. In time she recovered and is quoted as saying 'I adore yoga, but you have to be mindful when doing these things.'

And indeed, one of the main problems seems to be competitive practitioners who throw themselves into a practice without sufficient experience. 'The most common form of injury is the overzealous student', says Dr Loren Fishman, a spine specialist, yoga teacher and medical director of Manhattan Physical Medicine and Rehabilitation in an article in the *New York Times*. 'The second most common reason for injury is poor alignment, and that is usually crummy teaching.'

This hits on a raw spot in the yoga community. There is no formal accreditation of yoga teachers either here or in the US. That is to say there is not a centralised agency supervising the safety or certification of yoga instructors. The closest thing to regulation is found through non-profit, voluntary registers like the British Wheel of Yoga in the UK, The Independent Yoga Network, and the Yoga Alliance in the US and the UK. All of these organisations resist any kind of legally enforceable regulation claiming that yoga, as a spiritual enterprise, must be free from government interference.

Training for teachers can vary, and classes are so large in some studios that instructors cannot pay attention to what everyone is doing. In some classes, there are so many that not only can the teacher not see what everyone is up to, but students crash into each other. This is where the Iyengar method comes into its own. Iyengar teachers are rigorously trained and the whole practice is focused on proper alignment. Each pose is slowly entered with the help of props and adjustments are made. It is the safest practice of all. In fast, flowing yoga such as Ashtanga, you are far more likely to do yourself an injury, and in hot yoga or Bikram yoga, the heat can give you a false impression of how far you should push yourself, and you go beyond a safe range of motion.

And, indeed, the trend for what Americans term 'kick-butt' yoga – that is a vigorous aerobic workout taught by fitness instructors who might only have attended a weekend yoga workshop – means that injuries are also on the menu.

'Yoga is a good thing, so you tend to push yourself further than you would in a sport where you are more attuned to injury and afraid of injuries,' says Dr Michelle Carlson, an orthopaedic surgeon in Manhattan who specialises in arms and hands. The lesson seems to be that if any part of your body is protesting, then back off straight away. In the end, you have to take responsibility for your own body and 'listen to it'. A good teacher should always offer easier alternatives to any given pose for anyone not comfortable with the original.

The American Academy of Orthopaedic Surgeons (AAOS) believes that the rewards of basic yoga outweigh the potential physical risks, as long as you take care and perform the asanas in moderation according to your ability. To help minimise yoga-related injuries, it recommends the following:

1. Ask your doctor if you have any medical conditions or injuries before participating in yoga
2. Work with a qualified yoga instructor – ask about experience and credentials
3. Warm up thoroughly before a yoga session – cold muscles, tendons and ligaments are vulnerable to injury
4. Wear appropriate clothing that allows for proper movement
5. Beginners should start slowly and learn the basics first
6. Ask if you don't understand the instructions for a pose
7. Know your limits – do not try positions beyond your experience or comfort level
8. Find out which style of yoga will best suit your needs
9. Keep hydrated by drinking of plenty of fluids before class
10. Listen to your body

And my tip of the day is, if you're going to injure yourself, make sure it's a muscle or tendon you pull – they bounce back eventually. Do not tear a ligament – they don't stretch – and a damaged ligament means an unstable joint and then you're in trouble. And be aware of these zones: neck, knees, lower back and hamstrings. If any of them ever feel uncomfortable, back off. You are responsible for your own body.

All of this is of course commonsense. The bad

news is that some people will always have accidents or push themselves too far; the good news is that the benefits of yoga are widely agreed to outweigh the chances of injury (and that compared with other forms of exercise, yoga generates fewer and less costly insurance claims).

The other good news is that for many yoga-related injuries there are yoga-based solutions. Yoga Therapy is huge and is only just emerging as a discipline in itself. Briefly, yoga therapy is the adaptation of yoga practices for people with health challenges. It helps people manage their condition, reduce symptoms, restore balance, increase vitality and improve attitude. According to the International Association of Yoga Therapy, it is amongst the most effective complementary therapies for several common ailments, especially many chronic conditions that persist despite conventional medical treatment.

It comprises a wide range of mind/body practices, from postural and breathing exercises to deep relaxation and meditation. It aims for the holistic treatment of various kinds of psychological or somatic dysfunctions ranging from back problems to emotional distress. It has been shown to help patients recovering from injuries, surgery and illness, and is especially recommended for counteracting stress and depression.

Yoga Therapy is currently offered in the UK at a number of NHS hospitals and there are any number of private practitioners and workshops. The Complementary & Natural Healthcare Council, which is supported by the Department of Health, has established a voluntary register of yoga therapists.

Robin Munro, director of the Yoga Biomedical Trust which promotes the development of yoga therapy in the UK, has seen a huge growth in recent years and says that increasingly psychiatrists and GPs are referring patients to yoga therapists, and that there are lots of self-referrals too.

7

Breath of Life

One of the things I never envisaged doing before I took up yoga was sitting in a room full of other people learning how to breathe.

Bad Breath:
Breathing is something we don't think about until we can't do it very well, like when a fishbone becomes lodged in your throat or you run too hard for a bus. I once had a condition which was rather unkindly named *Globus hystericus* in medical jargon. I felt as though I had a tennis ball in my oesophagus and could neither breathe properly nor swallow. Naturally, I was fearing the worst, but after a lengthy and painful examination by a distinguished ear, nose and throat surgeon, I was told that apart from 'wonky sinuses' that there was no obstruction whatsoever – I just felt as though there was – hence the term 'hystericus'. Somewhat affronted, I thought the great man was being a trifle sexist until he assured me that men got it too. In fact, it's a pretty common stress-related symptom.

Since the body can go for many weeks without food,

and for days without water or sleep, but only a matter of minutes without air before life ceases, it seems extraordinary that most of us not only never think about the way they breathe, but also only use a fraction of our full breathing capacity. No wonder we all feel so tired the whole time. A combination of poor posture, stress and sedentary occupations mean that most people breathe by expanding only their upper chest when they inhale. This can result in an imbalance of oxygen to carbon dioxide resulting in hyperventilation, fatigue and sometimes dizziness.

To see how we should be breathing, you only need to look at a baby whose stomach expands and contracts naturally as it inhales and exhales. Proper breathing is governed by the movement of the diaphragm and should be full and rhythmic, the abdomen expanding as fresh air is drawn in through the nose and into the lungs. Deep abdominal breathing promotes a full exchange of air, keeping the oxygen/carbon dioxide ratio balanced. The inhalation brings energy into your body; the exhalation relaxes your body, expels the stale air and eliminates toxins. Proper breathing can tone up your entire system and enhance health and vitality. Most people use only a fraction of their lung capacity. They breathe shallowly, hardly expanding the ribcage and hardly drawing any oxygen in, and then wonder why they feel tired so easily.

Good Breath:

Yoga is all about breathing correctly; in fact, the breathing you learn in yoga probably revitalises you even more than practising the asanas. Indeed it is so important that a yogin – a master of yoga – measures his life not in years but in the number of breaths allotted for his lifetime. If he breathes hurriedly, he reasons, he squanders his time on earth. Breath control in yogic terms is called Pranayama where 'prana' means 'life force' or 'energy' and 'yama' means 'control' or the cessation of breath.

Pranayama is the fourth limb of the eight limbs or basic tenets of yoga and the pranayama breathing exercises that one does in yoga are the link between the physical and mental disciplines of yoga. The Yogis believe that prana circulates through the human body via a network of special channels called nadis (about 72,000 of them) criss-crossing the body and roughly equivalent to our network of nerves and blood vessels. The nadis are themselves governed by seven chakras (meaning wheels). These centres of energy are sited along the spine and blockages in the chakras can cause physical and mental problems. I talk at greater length about Prana and Chakras in Chapter 9.

Desmond Dunne, who wrote a book called *Yoga Made Easy* back in 1962, says that in a single day we breathe about 23,000 times. But the average person, especially a sedentary one, is still deprived of the optimal amount of oxygen he or she needs to supply the brain and heart which makes them prone to far more infection than people who lead active, outdoor lives. As Jo Average reaches middle age, his lung tissues grow less elastic and years of improper breathing takes its toll. Uric acid tends to accumulate in the blood stream which often leads to the numerous vague complaints doctors hear every day about aches, pains and stiffness.

Breathing in yoga should generally be done through the nose – both inhalation and exhalation. Nostril hairs filter dust particles and the mucous lining helps to kill germs. As air travels up the nasal passages it is warmed, ready to be taken into the lungs. These benefits are lost if you breathe through your mouth. It also helps not to look like the village idiot.

What interested me when I began practising yoga was just how important the breath is for actually getting you deeper into the postures. Having been dismissive when first invited to 'practise breathing' – yeah, I can do that – been doing it for years, was my ignorant attitude – I suddenly began to see the point when doing a forward bend. I had managed to grasp the point about hinging from the hips rather than just curving my spine but was still having difficulty in comfortably reaching my toes with straight legs. It was only when my teacher exhorted to me to take a deep breath in and then lean further forward on the exhalation that I found myself magically getting further down and forward just with the aid of breath.

Correct breathing also acts as a natural tranquilizer to the nervous system. The advice to 'take a deep breath' when someone is angry or agitated is sensible. The deeper you breathe, the calmer your mind becomes. Your breath is a safe, effective and free remedy for fatigue and all manner of mental and emotional instability.

Yogis of course have known this for centuries and have used the breath and breathing techniques to alter their state of mind. They didn't understand the science behind this, but now we do. When we are stressed, we breathe more rapidly. This leads to a build-up of oxygen in the bloodstream and a corresponding decrease in carbon dioxide, which in turn upsets the acid-alkaline balance (the pH level) of the blood. This condition, known as respiratory alkalosis, can result in nausea, dizziness, confusion and anxiety.

In contrast, slowing the breath raises the carbon dioxide level in the blood which nudges the pH level back to a less alkaline state. This engages the parasympathetic nervous system which calms and soothes us in a number of ways including telling the vagus nerve to secrete acedtylcholine, a substance that lowers the heart rate.

In addition to influencing our quality of life, our life span is also dictated by the rhythm of respiration. The ancient yogis noticed that animals with a slow breath rate such as elephants and tortoises have long life spans, whereas those with a fast rate such as birds, rabbits and dogs live for far fewer years. From this, they realised the importance of slow breathing for increasing the human lifespan. Since respiration is directly related to the heart, a slow rate keeps the heart better nourished.

Yoga teachers will often tell you to 'watch your

breath', especially when in Savasana, the corpse-like pose you adopt to relax at the end of a practice. When you can focus your attention exclusively on your breath (an excellent way of stopping the internal chatter that goes on in our heads all day long), you are then in a good place for meditation, about which more later.

There are various breathing techniques used by yogis. In these, four aspects of breathing are utilised: inhalation (Pooraka); exhalation (Rechaka); internal breath retention (Antar Kumbhaka); external breath retention (Bahir Kumbhaka). The most important part of pranayama is actually the breath retention but this is advanced stuff and therefore more emphasis is placed on correct inhalation and exhalation at first in order to strengthen the lungs before Kumbhaka.

There are three basic types of breathing which affect the different areas of your lungs.

Clavicular breathing is the most shallow and worst possible type, using the upper lobes of the lungs. The shoulders and collarbone are raised while the abdomen is contracted during inhalation. Maximum effort is made, but a minimum amount of air is obtained. This is how most people breathe most of the time – especially women.

Thoracic or *Intercostal breathing* utilises the middle lobes of the lungs by expanding and contracting the rib cage. It expends more energy than abdominal breathing and is often associated with physical exertion when the body needs more oxygen.

Abdominal (or *diaphragmatic*) in which the stomach rises and falls uses the lower lobes of the lungs. This is the most natural and efficient way to breathe (like a baby) but most adults have lost the natural ability to do it due to tension, poor posture and lack of training.

Yogic Breath:
Full yogic breathing combines all three techniques and uses every part of the lungs. It is used to maximise inhalation and exhalation and is used to correct poor breathing habits and increase oxygen intake. It is useful in stressful and angry situations for calming the nerves. It is simple to practise: you inhale slowly through the nose, making the abdomen expand first like a balloon then moving the breath upwards through the rib cage (including the side ribs) and finally feel the air filling the upper chest. Then you exhale as slowly as you can through the nose, completely emptying the lungs. It takes practise to be comfortable with it, but it is really worth trying. The clincher for me was reading about a recent shipwreck disaster where one of the passengers who had to spend a gruelling amount of time in a lifeboat waiting for rescue was the only one to survive and remain sane. When asked about his luck, he replied that it wasn't down to luck so much as yogic breathing.

Control of breathing (or Prana) leads to control of the mind which is vital for concentration and meditation. Breath is a reflection of what is happening in your head. Each frame of mind will subtly alter your breath. It is not for nothing that people tell you to take a deep breath when you are nervous or angry. Any reader of crime thrillers will tell you that you know when a lunatic is behind you, ready to strike, by his ragged agitated breathing.

In most yoga practices, you will probably do alternate nostril breathing (Nadi Shodhana) where you inhale through one nostril, keeping the other closed and then exhale through the other nostril. Nadi means 'channel' or 'flow' and Shodhana means 'purification'. This also calms and balances the body and strengthens respiration although it makes me feel a bit dizzy when it is combined with Kumbhaka (breath retention).

The one I really like is Bellows Breath (Bhastrika) which is dynamic and energising abdominal breathing in which you inhale and exhale very fast through your nostrils so that your stomach pumps in and out like bellows. This is fabulously beneficial: it boosts metabolic rate, stimulates the liver, pancreas and spleen, tones the digestive system and, best of all, BURNS FAT. A variation of this is Kapalabhati breath, another cleansing breathing exercise in which you concentrate on a forceful exhale through your nostrils in quick succession – good for cleaning sinuses, clearing mucus and stimulating the entire respiratory system (have a handkerchief handy).

Ujjayi (victorious) Breath is a method of yogic breathing whereby you contract the back of your throat to slow down the breath which will make a hissing sound like steam being released from a radiator even with your mouth closed (which it should be). More poetically, it is sometimes referred to as 'ocean breath' likening the sound to the sea advancing and retreating. It can be used during asana practice and is good for increasing oxygen in the blood, reducing phlegm and strengthening the immune system. It's not the kind of thing you want to try in public for fear of sounding like Darth Vader and frightening people on the bus, but it is an effectively powerful way of breathing when you are doing vinyasa style yoga and is used in yoga therapy to calm the mind and soothe the nervous system.

Another kind of breath which you probably don't want to do in public is Bee Breath (Brahmari), where you make a humming sound like a bee as you exhale slowly through your nostrils. I say you don't want to do it in public, though it always strikes me as an effective way of terminating a conversation you don't want to be having, or bringing a boring meeting to a halt, especially since your eyes should be closed. If challenged, you declare that it's to help you overcome insomnia (which it does).

There are many other types of breath but I shall mention one more which is useful – the cooling breath (Sheetali) where you stick out your tongue and roll it up at the sides so it forms a tube. This practice cools the body and the mind as well. It can be used as a tranquilliser before sleep and gives you (much-needed in my case) control over hunger and thirst. Fortunately, I fall into the two thirds of the population that are able to roll their tongues in this fashion (about a third of people are genetically incapable of this but I am sure that those people are able to sit in lotus or put their feet behind their head to make up for it).

And of course breathing is the key to meditation – that elusive state of nirvana where you achieve bliss and enlightenment. Or not – if you're like me and can't even sit still in a lotus position. But, it is certainly a worthy goal, not least because new developments in neuroscience suggest that the ancient eastern practice of meditation might delay the ageing process by protecting our chromosomes from degenerating.

8

Unseen Forces

A part of yoga that I struggle with is the unseen forces. I have a friend, even more cynical than myself, who mockingly calls me a 'chakra-botherer' – a New Age version of a God-Botherer – just because I do yoga. But this couldn't be further from the truth: I am not a chakra botherer because I don't bother with chakras and, what's more, I don't think you have to.

What you probably do need to do if you practise hatha yoga is at least know what they are supposed to be. This is because they are an integral part of yoga and yoga teachers will mention them in the class in the same way as they talk about your hamstring muscles or your pituitary gland – as if they are real. I mean, I know what gnomes are, but I don't happen to think that they really exist – except in suburban gardens. Chakras do not come to light in autopsies, but it doesn't stop people believing in them and yoga teachers telling you to focus on them.

Prana is another word you need to know. In Vedantic philosophy, prana is the notion of 'life force' or 'breath of life'. It is comparable to the Chinese Chi or Japanese Ki. In yoga and Ayurveda, it is a central concept and is believed to flow through a network of invisible channels called Nadis. Its most subtle material form is the breath, but it is also to be found in the blood and semen. In Ayurveda, Prana is thought to suffuse all living forms and the sun is a source of pranic energy.

The Chakra is a concept originating in Hindu texts and is part of many philosophical and spiritual traditions, as well as many therapies. Its name derives from the Sanskrit word for 'wheel' or 'turning' and in traditional Indian medicine, there are seven primary chakras – whorls of energy or force centres – which are thought to exist in the etheric human body. 'Etheric' takes some explaining too, but briefly it is the invisible double of the human body and is a term favoured by Theosophists.

The seven chakras, each of which is associated with a different colour, are located along a central nadi called Sushumna, which runs alongside or in the Spine. They are placed at major branches of the human nervous system, beginning at the base of the spinal column and moving upwards to the top of the skull. Each chakra is believed to influence or govern bodily and mental functions near its region. The chakras are visualised as lotuses/flowers with a different number of petals in each chakra.

The seven primary chakras with their associated areas of influence and colours are:

1. The Base/root chakra (Muladhara) – ovaries, prostate: red
2. The Sacral chakra (Swadhisthana) – the coccyx – last bone in spinal cord: orange
3. The Solar Plexus chakra (Manipura) – navel area: yellow
4. The Heart chakra (Anahata) – heart: green
5. The Throat chakra (Vishuddha) – throat and neck: blue
6. The Third Eye chakra (Ajna) – pineal gland: indigo
7. The Crown chakra (Sahasrara) – top of head, 'soft spot' of newborn baby: white

In Western culture, the theory of the seven main chakras was popularised largely through the translation of two Indian texts and a resulting book by Sir John Woodroffe called *The Serpent Power*. The ideas contained in this book were developed by C.W. Leadbeater in his book *The Chakras*.

Because of the similarities in belief between the Chinese and Indian healing traditions, the notion of chakras was also blended into Chinese therapies such as acupuncture and shiatsu.

One of the most accessible ways of understanding abstract concepts like prana and chakras – even the concept of yoga itself – is by reading Iyengar's book *Light on Pranayama* (first published 1981). It's the sequel to *Light on Yoga*; the classic text on the practise of Hatha yoga. *Light on Pranayama* doesn't only deal with breathing techniques, but provides a comprehensive background of yoga philosophy and discusses the allied topics of Nadis, Bandhas, Chakras, Kundalini and the like.

Iyengar says: 'It is as difficult to explain Prana as it is to explain God. Prana is the energy permeating the universe at all levels. It is physical, mental, intellectual, sexual, spiritual and cosmic energy. All vibrating energies are prana. All physical energies such as heat, light, gravity, magnetism and electricity are also prana. It is the hidden or potential energy in all beings, released to the fullest extent in times of danger. It is the prime mover of all activity. It is energy which creates, protects and destroys. Vigour, power, vitality, life and spirit are all forms of prana.'

Prana flows through the Nadis – a network of several thousand invisible tubular channels most them starting around the heart and the navel. The equivalent in the real body would be arteries, veins, capillaries etc., but in what Iyengar calls 'the subtle body' they are channels for the flow of consciousness which connect at special points of intensity (chakras).

One would have to be a serious student of Ayurveda to fully understand this crucial but very complex system within the subtle body. Another very difficult concept which you may come across and I should just try to summarise is Kundalini.

On Kundalini, Iyengar says: 'Kundalini is divine cosmic energy. The word is derived from 'kundala'

meaning a ring or coil. The latent energy is symbol-
ised as a sleeping serpent with three and a half coils;
it has its tail in its mouth, which faces downwards. It
lies at the hollow base of the Sushumna, two digits
below the genital area and two above the anus. The
three coils represent the three states of mind (awake,
dreaming, and deep sleep). There is a fourth state,
combining and transcending the others, which is represented by the last half-coil. It is attained in
Samadhi' (inner awareness achieved through meditation).

In Kundalini yoga, the object is to raise this
energy (that was unleashed in creation) through the
chakras from the base of the spine to the crown
chakra resulting in union with God or the Divine.
The Bihar school of yoga, for example, performs
various practises such as asanas and pranayama to
purify the nadis, meditation specific to each chakra
and finally the raising of the Kundalini itself.

Kundalini has been identified with cosmic energy
and with sexual drive. The end of Kundalini's
journey, union with the highest chakra, is Samadhi.
The techniques used to arouse the force of
Kundalini are likened in the literature of Hatha yoga
to the effect of beating a snake with a stick. They are
very physical, and include movements such as
bouncing up and down on the buttocks.

I have heard some hair-raising stories of people who
don't know what they're doing, trying to raise their

Kundalini without a proper, experienced guru to guide them through it. The various very physical practises that are involved can be dangerous for anyone who is less than stable to begin with. My yoga teacher met someone in India who couldn't the shake off the idea that his cat spirit had jumped into one of his open chakras. Quite a few people like this end up in mental asylums so it's not something I'm thinking of giving a go. Even Jung cautioned against it:

'One often hears and reads about the dangers of yoga, particularly of the ill-reputed Kundalini yoga. The deliberately induced psychotic state, which in certain unstable individuals might easily lead to a real psychosis, is a danger that needs to be taken very seriously indeed. These things really are dangerous and ought not to be meddled with in our typically Western way. It is a meddling with Fate, which strikes at the very roots of human existence and can let loose a flood of sufferings of which no sane person ever dreamed. These sufferings correspond to the hellish torments of the chönyid state...' C. G. Jung, Introduction to *The Tibetan book of the Dead*

Like the Doshas which I came across in India, it is all fascinating stuff to read about and try to understand. However, I have difficulty with belief systems which are not validated by science and it seems to me that the average student of Hatha yoga does not have to be concerned with ancient philosophies in order to feel the benefits of a yoga practice. Personally, I'd rather spend my time looking for unicorns than chakras; there's probably more chance I'll find them.

9

Meditation: Out of Your Mind

If, like me, the idea of some patchouli-scented, hippy-dippy, new-agey journey sends you running for the hills, or more likely the wine cellar, then, also like me, you are going to shy away from the whole idea of meditation But, hear me out.

Yoga – which I have now embraced – is doing a kindness to your body; that much we know. How about doing a service to your mind? Because that's what I choose to see meditation as – giving your mind a break, giving it a much needed rest. All day long (and often for part of the night) we are chattering to ourselves – worrying, wondering, plotting, analysing, agonising… planning the future, regretting the past, thinking about lunch… ceaseless, often pointless chatter. This is what the Buddhists called the 'monkey mind' – never still, always leaping about, and always babbling nonsense. And it is this monkey mind that needs to be subdued and tamed because thoughts are the barriers to the meditative state.

Before I did any yoga, I was never interested at all in meditation, even though I could see that if you just sit or lie still in one corner of the day and focus on your breath – just that – for as long as you possibly can, chasing away the random stuff that comes knocking on the mind's door, then you can begin to appreciate how mastery of this ancient art might be wonderfully beneficial, calming and rejuvenating. Why is this?

Let's start with the brain. Our brains are the result of the interaction between our genes and our experiences. Genes predispose you to things and experiences then wire up the brain. Nowadays we know about the enormous plasticity of the brain – it can be changed by behaviour. If, for example, you learn a new language or learn to play a new musical instrument, your brain will respond by creating new neural pathways to accommodate the new information it is receiving. You can also train your brain to abandon old neural pathways in favour of new ones – this is the basis for cognitive therapy.

In Chapter 3, I have already discussed some of the benefits on the brain of physical yoga including lowered blood pressure, mood enhancement, stress reduction, memory improvement and psychological equanimity. But, as you would expect, there is now a whole tranche of scientific research into what exactly happens to the brain when you meditate. This relatively new science called contemplative neuroscience is gaining more credibility and, importantly, more funding for research. In the U.S. the National Institutes of Health has upped its grants in complementary and alternative medicine ($300 million in 2007, to an estimated $541 million in 2011) and has helped establish new contemplative science research centres at Stanford University, Emory University, and the University of Wisconsin – the new home of the world's first brain imaging lab with adjacent mediation room.

One of the more recent studies has even more exciting implications – meditation can delay ageing. Yay! Now that really caught my attention. An extensive study co-ordinated by neuroscientist Clifford Saron of the Centre for Mind and Brain at the University of California has been conducted at a US Buddhist retreat in northern Colorado – the Shambhala Mountain Centre – where visitors meditate in silence for up to ten hours a day, emulating the lifestyle that monks have chosen for centuries. Saron's team advertised in Buddhist publications for people willing to spend three months in an intensive meditation retreat and choose 60 participants. Half of them attended in the spring of 2007 while the other half acted as a control group. Saron's team built a hi-tech lab in a dorm room beneath the Shambhala centre's main hall, enabling them to subject participants and controls to tests at the beginning, middle and end of each retreat, and worked with a 'village' of consulting scientists who each wanted to study different aspects of the meditators' performance.

People who meditate regularly will report on enhanced well-being but up until now it has been just hearsay. Now, a new generation of brain-imaging studies and rigorous clinical trials means that scientists are beginning to compile evidence that rather than simply being a feel-good spiritual experience, meditation could have long-term implications for physical health. One result in particular garnered at Shambhala has exciting implications: mediation protects caps called telomeres on the ends of our chromosomes. Telomeres limit the lifespan of cells and every time a cell divides, its telomeres get shorter, unless an enzyme called telomerase builds them back up. When telomeres get too short, a cell can no longer replicate, and ultimately dies. People with shorter telomeres are at greater risk of heart disease, diabetes, obesity, depression and degenerative diseases and they die younger.

In the Shambhala project, neuroscientists found that meditators had significantly higher telomerase activity than the control group, suggesting that their telomeres were better protected. It's early days, but the hope is that meditation and other psychological factors can slow or even reverse cellular aging and cognitive decline.

Other physical benefits of meditation which are more easily established are the lowering of blood pressure, the boosting of the immune response in vaccine recipients and cancer patients, and even the faster healing of psoriasis. In clinical settings it is used as an effective method of stress and pain reduction.

So how can focusing the mind have such astonishing physical effects? You only have to consider the extraordinary feats of Eastern yogis, fakirs and shamans who, apart from famously sitting on beds of nails, can suspend their breath for long periods of time and stop the beating of their hearts. Examples and studies of people voluntarily entering a state of suspended animation, in countries such as India, West Africa and Egypt, also abound. There are records from the 19th century of Indian yogis suspending their breathing or decreasing it to such a degree as to be undetectable, and, if these accounts are to be believed, then allowing themselves to be buried alive for days at a time.

'We all know that if you engage in certain kinds of exercise on a regular basis, you can strengthen certain muscle groups in predictable ways,' says Richard Davidson at the University of Wisconsin where his research team has hosted scores of Buddhist monks (who meditate for 10 hours a day) and other meditators for brain scans. 'Strengthening neural systems is not fundamentally different. It's basically replacing certain habits of mind with other habits.' In spite of the active participation of the Dalai Lama in arranging for Tibetan monks to travel to American universities for brain scans, Davidson points out that it is not a project about religion. 'Meditation is a mental activity that can be understood in secular terms.'

We now know from brain-imaging studies that meditation triggers active processes within the brain causing physical changes to the structure of the regions involved in learning, memory, emotion regulation and cognitive processing. According to scientist Charles Raison, who studies mind-body interactions at Emory University in Atlanta: 'Our understanding of the brain-body dialogue has made jaw-dropping advances in the last decade or two'. This is true especially in the field of how the body responds to stress. Meditation seems to be effective in changing the way that we respond to external events which produce stress. The body produces less of the stress hormone cortisol, and generally alters participants' psychological state so that they perceive the world as less threatening.

Most of the world's great religions have a meditative tradition. Forms of meditation were used in ancient Greece, among early Christians and in Judaism, but the practice in the West did not become widespread until the 1960s, driven by a surge of interest in eastern culture. Core meditation techniques have been preserved in ancient Buddhist texts and it is Buddhist meditation techniques which have become increasingly popular in the wider world for people chasing the two paramount mental qualities that arise from meditative practice identified by The Buddha: serenity and insight. Others describe it as finding the spiritual essence that resides in us all. Famous meditators are as diverse as Nick Clegg, William Hague, Madonna and Bob Marley; though they have kept their insights to themselves, thank god. Talking of which, if a book called *The Yoga of Jesus* by Paramahansa Yogananda is to be believed, then Jesus too was keen on meditation.

For me, meditation is a mystery – one, admittedly, that I haven't tried very hard to crack until now. The type of meditation taught by yoga requires preparatory disciplines which can only be learned through deep and protracted concentration where you focus exclusively upon one fixed point, often a body part or the 'third eye' in the forehead, or mantra. Once you can do that, you are ready to meditate and instead of staying with one point of focus, you can then let your mind relax – provided you stick to positive and constructive thoughts. The Yogis strive to achieve what they call 'Samadhi' which is variously described as a state of super-consciousness or infinite bliss. For Westerners, a more realistic goal is to learn to control and subdue negative thinking and gain self-knowledge.

An interesting article in the *Guardian* some years ago by Hazel Curry points out that the word 'Meditation' indicating deep thought is confusing. In fact, the whole point of it is not to think at all – to have a still mind with no thoughts whatsoever. She says it's about learning how to stop constantly thinking of things that worry you. We all panic about the future the whole time, when what we should be focused on is living in the present.

Desmond Dunne answers the charge that many negative-thinking sceptics like me would want to put to meditators – that of egotistical self-absorption. He says on the contrary, your enhanced insight into yourself will give you a greater understanding of others and that your relationships will become warmer and less judgemental: 'The self-knowledge brought about by systematic meditation will first become the basis for greater self-reliance and self-confidence and later will help improve every human equation of which you are a part. Through meditation you will gain a sense of perspective that will enable you to view the world around you objectively, to accept hard facts, gauge the good and the bad at their correct value, and so never again allow yourself to be weighed down with a sense of impotence or defeat. Similarly, there will be no room in your heart for envy, jealousy, resentment or hatred, since all these emotions stem from weakness, insecurity and fear. Instead, you will experience fresh inner strength which will be your balance wheel the rest of your life.'

Ed and Deb Shapiro, the award-winning authors of the book *Be the Change: How Meditation can transform you and the world* with forewords by the Dalai Lama and Robert Thurman, ask in the *Huffington Post* why something as simple as sitting still and watching our breath evokes panic, fear and even hostility. And it's true that there is something just so smug and irritating about people who claim meditation solves everything. As irritating as people who won't touch a grain of wheat or a blob of fat. But the Shapiros make some good points in their book for the uninitiated. The reasons they hear why people find it hard to meditate or just won't try are these:

I don't have time
I find it uncomfortable to sit still for so long
My mind won't stop thinking; I can't relax
There are too many distractions

I don't see the benefit
I'm not good at it
It's all just weird New Age hype

Pretty well all of these chime with my own objections. Their entirely reasonable response that you only have to try it and then stick with it for a while (in Japan it can take 12 years to learn how to arrange flowers...) to see the benefits. They also claim it's impossible to fail at meditation: 'even if you sit for 20 minutes thinking non-stop meaningless thoughts, that's fine...there are as many forms of meditation as there are people who practise it.' Make friends with meditation, they say, and it's a companion for life.

Of all types of meditation, I am most drawn to Transcendental Meditation, the movement popularised by Maharishi Mahesh Yogi and practised by an estimated five million people around the world. I like the fact that by far the bulk of scientific research on meditation is done on TM. I also like the fact also that I can concentrate on a word (a mantra, which is also a sound) instead of having to visualise something, which you are often asked to do whilst meditating and which I find incredibly difficult. No, I can't visualise my red chakra or my seventh vertebrae of pranic energy swilling around my third eye. You either think in pictures or words – and my bag is words. I am the kind of infuriating television viewer who is addicted to crime serials but never quite gets what is going on and has to keep asking the person next to me (who longs to commit some real-life crime as a result). This is why I am a competent crime novel reviewer but an incompetent crime film reviewer.

Anyway, back to TM. In 1950s India, the Maharishi's technique, based, as I have said, on using a mantra as a vehicle to attain a quiet mind, was presented in religious and spiritual terms as derived from the Hindu God Krishna and practised by Buddha. In the 1960s, the Maharishi began to promote his methods by going on a series of world tours which attracted celebrity attention, notably the Beatles et al. The result was that TM went global and attracted as much ridicule as it created followers.

By the 1970s, however, the emphasis changed to scientific verification in an effort to improve its image and to disassociate itself from any religious belief. There has been ongoing research since the first studies were conducted at the UCLA and Harvard and published in *Science* and the *American Journal of Physiology* in 1970 and 1971. In the 1990s the focus of the research has been the effects of TM on cardiovascular disease.

Now there are hundreds of such studies independently conducted at universities throughout the world and published in scholarly journals detailing the various benefits of TM. These are said to include decreases in stress hormones like cortisol, decreases in muscle tension and blood pressure, increases in memory and concentration, reduction of cardiovascular risk factors and the stabilization of the autonomic nervous system.

Brain wave activity, recorded in EEG research,

shows that the electrical output of the front and back parts of the brain as well as that of the two hemispheres becomes more synchronised. In science-speak, the brain becomes more 'coherent'. This has in important effect reported by several people I know who practise TM. They say it helps them think more clearly and to focus more effectively.

All this sounds great but the real reason I want to try it is that I have a couple of very sensible friends who swear by it. And the more they tell me that even I will be able to do it and will love it, the more I itch to prove them wrong. That, and the fact that a study quoted in the *Journal of Neuroscience* discovered that the biological age of a TM group (average age 50) using standard measures of aging was, on average, 12 years less than their actual chronological age… Sir John Harvey-Jones, TV's Trouble-shooter, agreed: 'TM has helped me avoid going too far down the Victor Meldrew route'.

Before I actually sign up for the programme, I go to see Nigel Barlow, a well-known speaker and writer based in Oxford and long-time TM practitioner and teacher. Nigel is a former barrister (wrong career choice) who describes himself as a creative thinker who has inspired many individuals and companies around the world to re-think their lives and businesses. His books include: *Batteries Included! – Creating Legendary Customer Service,* and *Re-Think: How to think differently.*

Nigel looks reassuringly normal (i.e. no flowing beard or penetrative eyes) and tells me he was dragged along to a TM lecture by a friend whilst studying law at Oxford in his early twenties. When he first meditated, he says, 'it was like coming home. I thought I know this – this is familiar; safe and complete.' What he liked about it was that you just meditated (no big deal, twice a day for 20 minutes is recommended) and then you get on with life. 'It's like brushing your teeth.' Except that, unlike brushing his teeth, it helped him to stop worrying and to pass the exams he hadn't worked very hard for. 'Even after two weeks, I had a new ability to focus and to be centred. The meditation was like recharging your batteries – I had so much energy afterwards.'

He too is impressed by the research now done on meditation, which points to enormous mental, physical and emotional benefits. 'Physically, it puts you in a much more relaxed state than deep sleep; the mind settles down and the body settles down and it is an incredibly deep state. However, it's not a substitute for sleep, and unlike when you sleep, you are totally aware and awake throughout. For instance, I often meditate on a train, but I can still produce my ticket when asked.

'There is the delusion that meditation is very difficult, but it's not difficult. It's a fundamental piece of knowledge that got lost but you are taught a simple technique to get there and everyone, from all walks of life, over the age of ten can do it. It's effortless.'

One of the benefits of TM is that after meditation you feel rested and energetic – it's not like coming out of a doze and feeling groggy. Also, your reaction time is measurably faster afterwards which is why it's popular with pilots and sportsmen – many of whom Nigel has taught. 'There is a common misconception that you have to clear your mind of thoughts when you meditate, but that just makes you agitated (witness Elizabeth Gilbert's tortuous attempts to meditate in her best-selling book *Eat, Pray, Love*). But in TM, you don't do that – you don't have to try – it's a natural process – like speaking. It's a natural human ability.'

TM, he adds, combats fatigue and insomnia. 'Sleeping patterns generally get better. There is some important research on this called Recovery from Sleep Deprivation. People have got off medication and tranquillizers after meditation and a lot of doctors now prescribe TM to patients. In the U.S., the National Institute of Health has funded $25 million research on TM, especially in relation to heart complaints in African-Americans (who suffer from this four times as much as whites).

How does it differ from other forms of meditation, I wondered. 'It's absolutely not mindfulness', says Nigel. 'Mindfulness involves a degree of control and effort and anything involving control is not so beneficial. You a given a mantra in TM and that is the tool that takes your mind down and down until you're beyond thinking and in a state of inner fulfilment which, for want of a better word, is bliss. And when you come out, your mind is clear and charged – you are more intelligent and creative. With other techniques, using visualisation for example, you have to make an effort to clear your mind and that's very difficult. Your mind moves about naturally seeking the next stimulating thing or new sensation, and you don't try to stop that in TM.'

He then tells me about some success stories, in particular his involvement with the David Lynch Foundation of which he is justly proud. David Lynch is the film director who makes pretty dark scary films like *Mulholland Drive* and *Eraserhead*, but what most people don't know is that he is a long-time TM practitioner and has started his foundation to raise funds to teach TM to children at risk: from street kids or those in war zones, to military personnel who suffer from post traumatic stress disorder, to prisoners, to those in homeless shelters, to everyone who needs it. The success rate has been astonishing and it's probably worth quoting part of David Lynch's message:

> In today's world of fear and uncertainty, every child should have one class period a day to dive within himself and experience the field of silence – bliss – the enormous reservoir of energy and intelligence that is deep within all of us. This is the way to save the coming generation.
>
> I have been 'diving within' through the Transcendental Meditation technique for over 30 years. It has changed my life, my world. I am not alone. Millions of other people of all ages, religions, and walks of life practice the technique and enjoy incredible benefits.

Tell me more about bliss, I beg, resolving to sign up immediately, whilst suspecting that I will be the only one in the history of the TM movement who can't find it. Nigel laughs: 'It's like trying to describe eating a strawberry to someone who's never had one.'

10

I Try TM

I arrive at a terraced house in a city not far from where I live in the country and am greeted by my teacher, a nice, jolly lady who I will call Sheila. She had forgotten I was coming which was a good start and insisted on putting on some makeup before giving me my introductory session. She and her husband, Martin, have been teaching TM for donkey's years and between them have taught over a thousand people. Immediately, I have to ask if any of them were disappointed or couldn't do it. The answer is no, everyone can do it. Already I know I'll be the exception.

The house is reassuringly normal, apart from several pictures of the Maharishi dotted about which inevitably look rather tacky and cultish. All those Indian guru pictures seem to look like this and if you go to any of the temples, either here or in India, they are monuments of kitsch, so very different from the great cathedrals of Europe. One thing I am clear about is that I do not want to join a cult.

My introductory lecture is just to outline the benefits of TM, which I have already researched. We fix a date for the course itself – four consecutive days for about an hour and a half. The first day is a one-to-one with Sheila in which there is to be a small ceremony and I will be given my mantra. Then I will be taught the techniques of meditation and by the end of the hour I will be meditating myself. The following three days, there will be other course members and we will just be going over basic principles and asking questions.

On day one I am very nervous and rather excited – will this really transform my life? I turn up at Sheila's house clutching a strange collection of objects I've been told to bring with me: an unused white handkerchief, six fresh flowers and three sweet fresh fruits. Oh, and a cheque. The fee structure is based on a sliding scale according to your individual salary, but millionaires will be delighted to hear that it is currently capped at £590.

The ceremony – the 'puja' as it's called – involves both Sheila and Martin chanting a prayer in Sanskrit and uses the handkerchief, flowers and fruit. I don't understand what it's all about but the mystery is part of the product in TM. The same goes for the mantra. I am not allowed to tell anyone what it is, or say it out loud, and Sheila is evasive when I ask her how it's chosen. The point is you are supposed to feel that everything is very special. I don't mind, as long as it works.

As soon as the ten minute ceremony is over, Sheila tells me my mantra. It is a two-syllable sound that means nothing to me and when I ask how it's spelt or what it means, she smiles mysteriously. Clearly, I am a bit of a nuisance, but I've made no bones about the fact I'm a journalist. I'm told that I mustn't spell out here either my mantra or the techniques as to how to meditate so I'll respect that, but suffice it to say that there is literally nothing to it – which, I have to admit, is disappointing. I ponder this as I close my eyes and prepare to meditate for the very first time.

My research has informed me that meditation is a form of concentrated attention in which the mind is turned inward and focused on a single point of reference. This is achieved by uttering the mantra, a word given to the student during the initiation ceremony which is chanted silently over and over. The aim is to empty the mind of thoughts, feelings and fantasies, not by blocking their intrusion, which is impossible, but by observing them as they intrude and then always returning to the central task of attending to the mantra. In this way a state of inner peace is achieved.

With practise, it is said, the mind can transcend thought, is no longer bound by feelings or fantasies, and experiences 'awareness of itself alone'. Hence 'transcendental' meditation. In the Upanishads, this transcendence is a conscious state where 'the sun does not shine, the moon does not give light, the fire does not burn…' This brings to mind a line in T.S. Eliot's Burnt Norton, one of the Four Quartets in which he talks of 'the still point of the turning world'. How wonderful to be there, I think.

So I sit as still as I can for fifteen minutes with my eyes closed, repeating my mantra to myself while the teacher bustles about. Outside in the street, I can hear people talking, getting into cars and so on. I think about that for a while, then I worry about what I look like with my eyes closed and then I try to get back to the mantra. Soon I start to fidget and then everything starts to itch so has to be scratched. After five minutes, I am fatally bored and wonder when I can open my eyes again. Then I begin to feel really cross that I've spent all this money on merely being given a sound and told to think it to myself. After ten minutes, though, I settle down. I become unaware of my breathing and realise that I'm sitting very still. Sometimes, I remember to say my mantra, sometimes my thoughts drift off.

Finally, Sheila says I can open my eyes. 'You did really well,' she says. 'How do you feel?' 'Tired', I say, and 'still'. I don't think I have ever closed my eyes for such a long time without actively trying to fall asleep. I feel relaxed but I am certain that I haven't 'transcended'. 'When am I going to feel the promised bliss?' I ask. 'You may experience the bliss later,' she says, 'it doesn't have to be in the meditation. You may find you just feel utter peace and contentment, even if only for a second or two, at any time'. I have to be satisfied with this.

I go home, promising to practise for the recommended 20 minutes every morning and every evening. Sheila says I will probably feel tired at first, but the idea is that meditation is restorative so that you can go about your day with energy. That night, I break my pledge straight away. I am supposed to meditate before eating but when I get home, everyone is having a pre-dinner drink and obviously I do too. Before I long I am eating and then, overcome with remorse at about 10pm I try to meditate but fall soundly asleep on my beanbag. I go to bed grumpy – this is hopeless. I knew I wasn't cut out for it.

The next morning is more successful. Before I get up, I sit up in bed and meditate. This time, I feel myself becoming still and slowing down much more quickly. My hands, which are in my lap become tingly, then numb. I am greatly encouraged by this as, according to Sheila, it shows I'm meditating correctly. When I finally glance at the clock, I realise 40 minutes have gone by – this is astonishing. Normally, I cannot be still for more than a minute or two. I have exceeded my goal by 20 minutes without being aware of it. I text Sheila the good news.

At the next group session, we all talk about our experiences. Another woman there, about my age, has evidently had no success at all. She says she can't stop thinking and that she feels pressurised by having to find the time to meditate twice a day when there's so many other things to get on with. I know exactly how she feels and sympathise. The candidate who seems to be doing the best is a ten year old girl, the daughter of meditators. Children from the age of ten can do TM and often find it much easier than the adults. They probably don't come loaded with the same kind of expectations.

We are told that when thoughts interrupt the mantra and the meditation, not to worry. You just need to observe them – they are stress releasers – and then get back to the mantra. The whole point of TM is that it is supposed to be absolutely effortless which is why anyone can do it.

At the end of my course, these are my feelings about the TM experience:

It is a novel experience for most people to try to sit still and switch off a couple of times a day with their eyes closed. It has got to be beneficial whether or not you 'transcend'. Apparently, the stillness achieved during meditation also slows down the metabolism of the body providing a deep state of rest which is rejuvenating, especially for the nervous system.

I agree that concentration is the key to a disciplined mind and that a concentrated mind is a powerful mind. Although it sounds contradictory, a concentrated mind is also a relaxed mind. It's a worthwhile aim just to try to focus on one thing (like a mantra) for a small amount of time each day. After all, the firm control of the senses is the yoga of the mind and since it took me a while to get into the yoga of the body, so I shall give over some time to getting into the yoga of the mind.

The hush-hush secrecy of it all is nonsense but we love to feel they are part of something mystical and special. There is a cultish feel to it all that is completely unnecessary. The truth is (as anyone can find out on the internet) is that your mantra is given you according to age and gender and that thousands of other people will have the same one as you. But, so what? A mantra is as useful as anything else for the mind to latch on to when it is trying to rest.

The fees charged are pretty hefty for something that can be learned by anyone at any time. Many TM teachers have become concerned about the cost and have left the organisation to offer instruction on their own. On the other hand, if you have forked out a month's wages, you might be more inclined to give it a proper go.

The benefits are pretty well documented in the areas of decreased blood pressure, lowered stress, cholesterol, and anxiety. I don't find this surprising since the stillness achieved during meditation also slows down the metabolism of the body which provides a deep state of rest and rejuvenates the body, especially the nervous system. Certainly, it leaves you feeling more relaxed and more content so that's got to be good. One of TM's most contentious claims in the early days was that TMers could fly (yogic flying) and levitate. This claim, having been subjected to ridicule, has been quietly dropped.

The celebrity endorsements (Donovan, The Beatles, Mia Farrow etc.) have been very beneficial to the global movement though, sceptic that I am, I distrust everything celebrities do. So, I guess it works both ways.

Worryingly, there are support groups for ex-TMers who are disenchanted not only with the claims made by TM, but also the money made by the organisation (which is supposed to be a non-profit organisation). Many of these claim that the same benefits accrue from listening to relaxing music or doing relaxation exercises. John Lennon fell out with the Maharishi and wrote a song 'Sexy Sadie' about his allegedly materialistic ways (gold Rolls Royce etc). However, you only have to look on the internet to find massive endorsement of the technique itself. In other words, there is only way to find out – do it yourself and see.

The Maharishi believed that the spiritual wellbeing of the world would be transformed if everyone spent 20 minutes a day meditating. I think he was being optimistic; but on the other hand I can think of about a million people who might be a little less angry... Oh, and he founded a political party, The Natural Law Party, which fielded candidates in elections in several countries including the UK. It is now mostly defunct.

In America, there have been celebrated court cases over attempts to introduce TM into public schools. They have failed, although there are private TM schools. In the UK there is one affordable private school, the Maharishi School in Skelmersdale, Lancashire, where most of the teachers are TM-ers and the children incorporate two sessions of TM at the beginning and end of the day into the curriculum. The academic results there are impressive and the children are apparently markedly better adjusted and happy than their non TM peers.

Conclusion: I am going to keep meditating and see what happens. If it works for me, great; if it doesn't, I'll stop. But I am mindful that I need faith or conviction that I will achieve my goal; that I have to practise regularly; and that I have to practise over a substantial period of time. Only then, can I really judge the whole experience fairly.

11

Eating Like a Yogi

'Can one truly be a yogi and a foodie?' asks a mournful *Guardian* blogger. 'Is it possible to practise the five abstentions (of which absence of avarice is one) while still enjoying a cheeky little merlot? Can we respect all living things while mindfully necking a steak?'

Sadly, I think I know the answer to this one without even consulting the yogic texts. A real yogi, unlike me, does not think about what might be for lunch upon waking in the morning – no, he leaps out of bed and does a headstand. Neither does he start twitching with anticipation of a glass of chilled Chablis at around 5pm. A real yogi eats to live, rather than lives to eat…

In fact the really real yogis seem to exist on a diet of mung beans and rice – a concoction known as 'kitcheree' (I thoughtfully provide a recipe for this in an appendix). My yoga teacher Marilyn says that when some of the yoga teachers are on their teaching circuits around the world, they even take their own camping stoves with them to make kitcheree. So clean are their systems that they reject all other food.

Less obsessive yogis try to stick to a Sattvic diet

which in Ayurvedic terms means fresh, pure food including most fruits, vegetables, whole grains, legumes as well as fresh dairy products. Leftovers and stale food are strictly a no-no – these, along with meat, fish, eggs, onions, mushrooms, garlic, and alcohol are known as Tamasic, thought to lead to a diseased body and a dull mind. Then there arc the in-between foods known as Rajasic or stimulant substances like tea, coffee, chocolate and hot spices which should also be avoided.

Yogi Bhajan, the Kundalini master, encourages his students to drink and eat certain 'healing' items every day in order to feel young, light and healthy. Some of these are: chlorophyll, rice bran syrup, turmeric, almonds, pomegranate juice, sesame oil, whey and yoghourt.

Sattvic foods like these are fresh, preferably organic, easy to digest and 'not disturbing to the mind'. They should be chewed thoroughly and eaten slowly. Unlike in the McKay family, where 'we sit at the table and smack our food like a bunch of possums in a mulberry bush', as Dolly Parton once remarked of her own family's table manners.

The way Sattvic food is prepared is important too. The cook's state of mind should be positive and the food is best prepared with 'love and awareness' (rather than salivating impatience I suppose).

Iyengar claims it is the duty of an aspirant yogi to find out by trial and experience which kind of food is suitable for him whilst stating that the practice of yoga and pranayama changes the eating habits for the better.

What is most important, he says, is the state of mind of the eater. A tyrant with a disturbed mind may eat Sattvic vegetarian food and still remain Rajasic or Tamasic. Whereas noble characters may not be affected by the wrong type of food. No-one should eat while emotionally disturbed, which rules most of us out for most of the time.

What everyone seems to agree upon is that food should only be eaten when hungry and then in moderation. Yoga texts say that the stomach should be half filled with solid food, quarter with fluids and a quarter left empty for the free flow of breath.

It's only too easy to fill up your body, but what about emptying it out and cleansing it? People are usually pretty good about cleaning the outside of their bodies, but in yoga the insides are also important. There are many yoga cleansing practices and rituals that clean out different parts of the body, most of which need to be performed under the instruction of a qualified teacher. Some of them are so esoteric (to the western mind) that it is unlikely you will want to try them. To give you an idea, one of them used to clean out the stomach (Vastra Dhauti) involves swallowing a clean, disinfected piece of muslin cloth leaving a bit hanging out of the mouth. The cloth is then pulled out, presumably with some of your stomach contents clinging to it.

Many of the techniques designed to clean out internal organs involve drinking copious amounts of salted water which is then vomited up. Others involve the introduction such as oils and herbal concoctions through the anus or vaginal orifice in order to clean the lower part of the body. There seems to be a cleansing technique for every single part of your body from your nostrils (neti) to your lower intestines. There is even one to purify your mind. Many of them sound completely revolting but practitioners swear by them. I recall from my Ayurvedic retreat that Indians don't feel at all squeamish about asking you intimate questions about your bowel movements or any other body process for that matter. They regard a clean body, inside and out, as a prerequisite to a clean mind and finally a clean spirit.

All of this of course makes perfect sense but is slightly discouraging to those of us in the West who start to dribble at the thought of roast beef and all the trimmings.

In my personal quest to be more of a yogi and less of a glutton, I fixed to go to one of the Spa Resorts in Ko Samui, an island off Thailand, to follow one of their legendary detox programmes which scarily included do-it-yourself colon cleansing. I plumped for the semi-fast programme (three and a half days as opposed to seven days) because, being there for only a week, I very much wanted to sample the After-Cleanse menu at their Radiance Restaurant for a few days too.

Before I could embark on this, I was advised to do a 'pre-cleanse' at home which involved drinking two 'Liver Flush' drinks a day with two meals consisting only of vegetables and salads. I actually managed to do this and I have to say I rather enjoyed the Liver Flush drinks, as, presumably, did my liver. The drink, being a blended mixture of virgin olive oil, fresh lemon juice, 3-5 cloves of garlic, a knob of ginger, cayenne pepper and fresh orange juice is not to everyone's taste though. My 20-year-old daughter Isobel, with whom I was embarking on this adventure, took one taste, spat it out and absolutely refused to have any more. I think my curious early preferences for swigging cough mixture and chewing aspirins probably helped me get through it.

When we got to Thailand, true to form, Isobel lasted for only a day on her detox fasting programme – in fact she was rather sick afterwards for a couple of days – while I manfully completed my three and half days during which I had no food at all – only the liver fast drink and a variety of health supplements conducive to a) cleaning out the colon and b) helping you not to feel hungry. To my surprise, I felt extremely well on it – very light and energised – and could have gone on with the fast if it wasn't for the fact we weren't going to be there for a long time. And I kept overhearing how delicious the restaurant food was.

What I didn't care for was the procedure by which you cleaned your own colon every evening in the privacy of your bathroom with the help of a coffee enema kit and a hose (I'll spare you the details). However, I will include the interesting tip that floating stools (as opposed to those that sink) and yellow urine are signs that your colon is in good shape. Just to encourage us to cleanse our colons, we were treated to photographs of some of the gunk that came out of previous clients' bodies including horrific, squirming wildlife (I kid you not.)

We both enjoyed the daily yoga as well as fabulous Thai massage and a whole variety of other treatments ranging from reflexology to cupping. And, of course, after the fasting, I don't think I have ever been so pleased to see a plate of salad and raw vegetables as I was in the Radiance Restaurant, which lived up to its name. Interestingly, nobody remotely missed the absence of meat and fish, although one night Isobel and I daringly crept down to a beach restaurant and stuffed ourselves with prawns. Another good tip: try to resist the overwhelming urge to go and lie down after a heavy meal. Walking after you eat is the thing to do. It is a tremendous aid to digestion in that it helps move lymph fluid which contains toxins that need to be excreted.

What I have noticed in myself, and what yogis tell me, is that if you do practise yoga regularly, you do start to adopt a different attitude to food. Good fresh food and yoga go hand in hand. There are now several high-profile chefs in the United States who are also yogis and they are helping to shape a more enlightened attitude to food – not only what we eat, but where we get the food from and choices we make. One of them, interviewed recently in Yoga Journal, is Bryant Terry. He describes himself as an 'eco-chef' and food justice activist. 'Food justice' he defines as universal access to wholesome sustainable food.

Whilst a graduate student at New York University, he became interested in the detrimental effect of poverty and poor nutrition on communities. 'I saw that in many marginalized communities throughout the States, there was little access to healthy, affordable and culturally appropriate food, but there was a plethora of foods that were high in salt, sugar and fat', he says. 'Many of these communities did not have full-service supermarkets, and if they did, those markets would have very little fresh food and lots of processed junk, while the same stores in higher-income neighbourhoods would have lots of fresh produce.'

Terry writes food books and hosts cooking demonstrations with gift bags of fresh produce. He says that yoga was his career catalyst and has helped him see food as a means to help people make decisions that both serve their own and the wider world's best interests. Another celebrated raw foods chef, who was trained in the classical French tradition, is Matthew Kenney, owner and director of 105 degrees Academy in Oklahoma City. His Academy trains new chefs in the methods, tools, ingredients and philosophy of raw food cuisine, and he attributes his 15 year yoga practice with giving him the flexibility and openness that translates to the kitchen. Some of his best recipe ideas, he says, come to him after practising. 'Yoga opens you in the way you allow it to. It makes room for creativity that you otherwise wouldn't have.'

I should also mention drink. It goes without saying that yogis try not to drink alcohol. But they do drink water – lots of it – starting the day without fail with half a pint of tepid water with half a lemon squeezed into it to cleanse the system. Otherwise, it's herbal teas such as lemon balm, peppermint, chamomile and various health drinks like wheatgrass or green barley juice. In recent times, Gwynnie et al can't be seen without coconut water and anything to do with pomegranates is coolywool. The sandwich chain Pret a Manger has, I notice, introduced a 'Pure Pret Yoga Bunny' drink which involves carbonated water and various herbal infusions. Me? Well, I look forward to a yogic claret anytime soon.

Perhaps more important to know is how to drink water if you are doing any form of exercise, yoga included. It is vital to stay hydrated and it's not good enough to walk into class with a bottle of water and take a swig before starting – it will not hydrate you in time. Indeed, some yoga teachers do not approve of drinking water during the class. All that happens is you immediately sweat the water out and it is not absorbed into the body where it is needed.

The smart thing to do is to drink water hours before your class begins which gives your body time to absorb the water properly. During a typical yoga class you can lose between three and five pounds of water weight because of all the stretching which affects the way the kidneys work. Toxins will duly be released but you need to have water already flowing through the body in order to flush them out in sweat.

I remember when I went on my first safari in Africa,

all the tourists lugging water bottles around with them and taking frequent swigs because of the hot sun. After a while I noticed that our African guide never had any water with him however many hours we were out for in the sun and asked him about it. He said he never got thirsty on the safari outings because he had always drunk a lot of water hours earlier.

When the yoga class is over, you then need to start drinking water to re-hydrate – not just straight after the class, but also throughout the day – not too much at a time though. You can tell from the colour of your urine whether you are de-hydrated as it will be a dark shade of colour. Talking of urine, yogis following an Ayurvedic routine are sometimes encouraged to drink their own urine between the hours of 4am and 6am in the belief that the hormones ingested will facilitate a meditative state.

12

Gurus, Who Needs 'em?

In traditional India you feel a fool not to have a guru in the true sense of a spiritual teacher. Indeed, the Indians consider you to be 'an unfortunate orphan' without one. In the West, however, if you go around telling people that you have a guru you will be pigeon-holed as the type of person who hands out colourful leaflets in supermarkets car parks proclaiming the end of the world. Your guru will, according to most psychiatrists, be schizophrenic at best and dangerously psychotic at worst.

The yoga world is actually full of them, although it's debatable how many of them deserve the name. There are the self-styled gurus like the notorious Bikram Choudhury and cultish teachers like John Friend, but they are too busy making money to do much spiritual guidance.

B.K.S. Iyengar, who of course has guru status himself, says in his book *Light on Pranayama* that a guru is 'a teacher of sacred knowledge who removes the darkness of ignorance and leads his pupil towards enlightenment and truth. He is also one from whom we learn right conduct or under whom one studies how to lead a good life... the guru is the bridge between the individual and God.'

The etymology of the word guru is as follows: In Sanskrit, the syllable 'gu' means shadows or darkness; the syllable 'ru' means he who disperses the darkness or light. According to one of the Upanishads, 'because of the power to disperse darkness, the guru is thus named.' In the Yogic word, it is thought that when a student is ready, a guru will appear – he doesn't have to look for one.

To be a guru, therefore, it is not enough to have great knowledge, wisdom or authority. The main idea is that you use that wisdom to guide others. In Hinduism and other religions, finding a true guru is held to be the prerequisite for attaining self realization. In contemporary India, the guru has a more general meaning of teacher. In the West, a guru has come to mean anyone who acquires followers – and there's the rub. Anyone can acquire followers, and anyone can set themselves up as a guru.

Notable dubious gurus include Bhagwan Shree Rajneesh, also known later on as Osho 'the sex guru', famous for his vast fleet of Rolls Royces, promotion of sexual freedom and a bioterrorist attack in Oregon carried out by some of his followers. Another is Sathya Sai Baba, the Indian guru with a vast international following estimated at 50 million who worshipped him as a living god. Sai Baba was accused of sexually abusing boy disciples and claiming false miracles in his lifetime and, after his death in 2011, an enormous hoard of gold, silver, precious stones, 500 pairs of shoes, a haul of watches and masses of stuff generally unrelated to abstemious godly ones, was discovered at his private quarters.

Anthony Storr, a British professor of psychiatry, argues in his book *Feet of Clay: A Study of Gurus*, that these kind of phoney gurus routinely share common character traits. They are, he says, likely to be loners and often suffer from a mild form of schizophrenia. Those who are authoritarian, paranoid and dictate how the lives of their followers should be led are the ones who are most likely to be dangerous.

Many academics and writers have drawn up checklists of warning signs to help identify false gurus and cults which do exploit and/or abuse their followers. Professor Eileen Barker, a sociology professor with special expertise in cults, lists the following traits in groups which could become dangerous as:

1. A movement that separates itself from society, either geographically or socially;

2. Adherents who become increasingly dependent on the movement for their view on reality;

3. Important decisions in the lives of the adherents are made by others;

4. Making sharp distinctions between us and them, divine and Satanic, good and evil, etc. that are not open for discussion;

5. Leaders who claim divine authority for their

deeds and for their orders to their followers;
6. Leaders and movements who are unequivocal-
ly focused on achieving a certain goal.

Clearly, in the West, we have a rather different attitude
to gurus and are sceptical of those who claim special
spiritual insights or new paths to salvation. Dr Georg
Feuerstein, a celebrated German-American Indologist
specialising in yoga has this to say in his book *The Deeper
Dimension of Yoga: Theory and Practice*:

'The traditional role of the guru, or spiritual teacher, is
not widely understood in the West, even by those pro-
fessing to practise yoga or some other Eastern tradition
entailing discipleship... spiritual teachers, by their very
nature, swim against the stream of conventional values
and pursuits. They are not interested in acquiring and
accumulating material wealth or in competing in the
marketplace, or in pleasing egos. They are not even
about morality. Typically, their message is of a radical
nature, asking that we live consciously, inspect our
motives, transcend our egotistic passions, overcome
our intellectual blindness, live peacefully with our
fellow humans, and, finally, realise the deepest core of
human nature, the Spirit.'

Some influential yogic gurus in the Hindu tradition in
the 20th century who conformed to these ideals
include:

Sadhguru Jaggi Vasudev (1957-), a yogi and mystic who founded the non-profit Isha Foundation offering yoga programmes around the world and involved in social and community work.

Sri Sri Ravi Shankar (1956-), the spiritual leader and founder of the Art of Living Foundation which tackles social problems. Also co-founder with the Dalai Lama of the International Association for Human Values, an NGO engaged in relief work and rural development.

Swami Sivananda (1887-1963): Served as a doctor in Malaya and was Founder of the Divine Life Society. Propagated Sivananda yoga in Europe and America.

Paramahansa Yogananda (1893-1952), Hindu spiritualist and yoga teacher who arrived in Boston in 1920 and is associated with Kriya yoga. Founder of the Self Realization Fellowship in Los Angeles in 1920 and author of the famous *Autobiography of a Yogi* (1946).

Swami Vivekananda (1863-1902), a key figure in introducing Vedantic philosophy and yoga to the Western world. He famously addressed the Parliament of World Religions in Chicago in 1893. Usually credited with being the father of modern yoga.

A.C. Bhaktivedanta Swami Prabhupada (1896-1977), founder of the Hare Krishna movement (the International Society for Krishna Consciousness) in

New York in 1965. He spread a movement based on Bhakthi yoga (yoga of devotion).

Maharishi Mahesh Yogi (1918-2008), popularised Transcendental Meditation in the 1960s.

Yogi Bhajan (1929-2004): Sikh yogi and master of Kundalini yoga (involving meditation and chanting). Established the 3HO (Healthy, Happy, Holy Organisation) in 1969 to further his missionary work. In the 1990s he created the International Kundalini yoga Teachers' Association.

T. Krishnamacharya (1888-1989): associated with early 20th century revival of yoga and guru to B.K.S. Iyengar, Sri K. Pattabhi Jois and T.K.V. Desikachar (his son). An early disciple was Indra Devi, sometimes called the First Lady of Yoga.

The importance of finding a guru is emphasised in Hinduism. One of the main Hindu texts, the Bhagavad-Gita, is a dialogue between God in the form of Krishna and his friend Arjuna, a Kshatriya prince who accepts Krishna as his guru on the battlefield prior to a battle.

The disciple of a guru is called a shisya or chela. Often the guru lives in an ashram or in a gurukula (the guru's household) together with his disciples. Hinduism proclaims that a guru is one's spiritual guide on earth and some believe that the guru can awaken dormant spiritual knowledge within his pupil (a process known as shaktipat).

Iyengar is unequivocal about the role of the proper guru: 'Initially, the guru brings himself down to the level of his pupil, whom he encourages and gradually lifts up by precept and example. This is followed by teaching adjusted to the pupil's fitness and maturity until the latter becomes as fearless and independent as his guru. Like a mother cat holding a blind and helpless kitten in her mouth, he first checks the movements of his pupil, leaving him with little initiative. In the next stage, he allows him the same freedom that a mother monkey does when her baby first releases its grip on her fur, for she keeps it close to her. In the first stage, the pupil is under the unquestionable discipline of the guru; in the second stage he surrenders his will completely. In the third stage, like the fish with unwinking eyes, he becomes both skilful and clean in thought, word and deed.'

'Pupils', he continues 'are of three categories – dull, wavering and intense or superior. The dull pupil has little enthusiasm, being sensual, unstable and cowardly. He is unwilling to shed his negative qualities or to work hard for self-realization. The second type of pupil is a waverer, equally attracted towards worldly matters as by the spiritual, sometimes giving weight to the one and sometimes to the other. He knows what is the highest good, but lacks courage and determination to hold on steadfastly. He needs strong treatment to correct his fickle nature of which the guru is aware. The intense or superior pupil has vision, enthusiasm and courage. He resists temptations and has no hesitation in casting off qualities which take him away from his goal. He therefore becomes stable, skilful and steady. The guru is always alert to find a way to guide his intense pupil to realise his highest potential until he becomes a realised soul (Siddha). The guru is always happy with his pupil, who may eventually surpass him.'

Gurus today:

Iyengar (born 1918), is probably the best known living guru we have. Born in southern India in the midst of the global influenza epidemic, his mother was stricken with it during the pregnancy and he suffered from health problems that plagued him for much of his childhood. Fortunately for him, his brother-in-law was the great guru Shriman Tirumalai Krishnamacharya, who helped create the hatha yoga style and invited Iyengar to move to Mysore where he took yoga lessons from the great man. At first, he was, he says 'an anti-advertisement for yoga', unable to touch his knees let alone his feet. But gradually under the disciplinarian regime of Krishnamacharya, he grew stronger and healthier, finally becoming a teacher himself.

His own experiences set him apart from other specialists at the time. He believed and indeed knew that anybody at all could benefit from yoga and he began to incorporate aids such as ropes, belts and blocks into yoga routines to help those who needed them to get into the poses. Many elderly people flocked to his classes and accomplished more than they could ever have expected. Iyengar was living testimony to the idea that yoga could benefit if not solve even the most serious health problems.

His followers soon included other famous Indians such as the philosopher J. Krishnamurti and the cardiologist Rustom Jal Vakil. It was Vakil's wife who introduced Iyengar to the classical violinist Yehudi Menuhin – one of his most famous students – who did much to introduce Iyengar to the West. In 1966 he published his seminal yoga text *Light on Yoga* which is still considered the bible of yoga around the world.

In later life, Iyengar divided his time between India and the West and in 1975 he established the Ramamani Iyengar Memorial Institute in Pune named after his late wife. This is still a key centre for the training of Iyengar instructors although there is said to be a five year waiting list. Two of Iyengar's children, daughter Geeta and son Prashant now continue his work there. You hear stories from people coming back from Pune that Iyengar (or Guruji as they call him) is such a demanding teacher that his initials B.K.S. should stand for Bang, Kick, Slap (as he makes his adjustments). But he has laughed this off, saying in one interview, 'The intensity of my approach makes the person who is dull become sharper... it's a disciplined subject. A casual attempt only gains casual results'.

The main guru of Ashtanga yoga, who died recently aged 93 in 2009, was K. Pattabhi Jois. In 1927 at the age of 12, Jois attended lecture and demonstration by

Krishnamacharya in the Jubilee Hall, Hassan, and became his student the very next day – although he kept it secret from his Brahmin family who professed no interest in yoga. In 1930 Jois ran away from home to Mysore to study Sanskrit and was later reunited with his guru. Jois developed his own style of hatha yoga incorporating a dynamic flow called vinyasa between poses which became known as Ashtanga, a high energy form of yoga. In 1948, he established the Ashtanga yoga Research Institute at Mysore which became a centre for pilgrimage for many westerners from the 1960s onwards.

T.K.V. Desikachar is the son of Krishnamacharya who left a civil engineering career to study yoga with his father. In 1976, along with another student A.G. Mohan, he established the Krishnamacharya Yoga Mandiram (KYM) to propagate the teachings of his father in Chennai, India. Today Desikachar is known as a world authority on yoga and the style he teaches is sometimes called Viniyoga. The KYM is a multi-departmental institution dedicated to teaching and researching yoga studies.

Indra Devi was born Zhenia Labunskaia in pre-Soviet Latvia. A friend of the Mysore royal family, she attended one of Krishnamacharya's demonstrations and asked him for instruction. At first he refused saying his school accepted neither foreigners or women, but she persisted and eventually Krishnamacharya started her lessons, subjecting her to strict dietary guidelines and a difficult schedule aimed at breaking her resolve. She met every challenge he imposed eventually becoming his good friend and exemplary student.

Devi wrote the first best-selling book on hatha yoga *Forever Young, Forever Healthy* published in 1953. In 1947 she moved to the United States living in Hollywood and attracted celebrity students like Marilyn Monroe, Elizabeth Arden, Greta Garbo and Gloria Swanson. Her style was gentler than Ashtanga and didn't employ vinyasa, though she used Krishnamacharya's principles of sequencing so that her classes followed a deliberate journey, and she combined asana with pranayama. She also added a devotional aspect called Sai yoga. She moved to Argentina in 1985 and her six yoga schools are still active in Buenos Aires.

Dharma Mittra, a practitioner of classical Ashtanga is known as the elder statesman of yoga in America – the teacher's teacher. Born in Brazil, Dharma began his studies with Swami Kailashananda known as Yogi Gupta who became his guru at an ashram in Manhattan. After intensive study of Ashtanga and Karma yoga, he was initiated as a sannyasi (one who renounces the world in order to realize God). In 1975, he opened the Dharma yoga Centre in Manhattan and in 1983 he started work on his famous poster of the 908 asanas (photographing himself in each pose) which can be seen hanging in gyms and ashrams throughout the world. His own series of poses is called Shiva Namaskar Vinyasa and is a five-level practice of poses which, in addition to physical benefits, focuses on the goal of self-realization. 'Everything is an act of adoration to the Lord', he says.

My thoughts on gurus? I tend to agree with my yoga teacher Marilyn who says: 'As far as I am concerned, there are no authorities on yoga – only individuals can determine their personal connection to the 'Great Spirit'. No 'gurus' or 'experts' can do it for anyone else.' The only guru she listens to is 'the inner guru' of which Amit and Banani Ray say in their book *Awakening the Inner Guru*: 'There is a subtle principle that resides within all of us, which is unborn and undying. It is a repository of infinite strength, wisdom, abundance and auspiciousness. It is bliss infinite and the giver of supreme happiness. It is the support-less, infinite sky of supreme wisdom. It is the silent witness of everything. It is neither male, nor female. It exists beyond all dualities. It is not bounded by time, space or conditions. This witnessing presence is pure and clear like the sky, luminous like the morning Sun. It is our inner Guru.'

Looks like I'm going to have to depend on that too. Gurus are thin on the ground where I live.

13

Men on Mats

When I go to my yoga class, my husband sometimes quips: 'Off to your physical jerks then?' It's meant to be funny, but there's also a note of sly contempt. If I said something along those lines when he was going to the gym, he'd be puzzled or annoyed. The fact is that men tend to think that yoga is for girls. It's not proper exercise, just a bit of stretching and faffing about with a touch of New Age spirituality thrown in for good measure. It reminds me of a story told in the louche ex-MP Tom Driberg's autobiography in which he picks up a huge, brawny Scots guardsman in a pub. After they've enjoyed themselves, Tom says to the soldier: 'Tell me Jock, what's a strapping lad like you doing with another man – I'd have thought you'd be out looking for lassies.' To which Jock replies: 'Och, no, girls are for sissies.'

It's true that three quarters or so of yoga practitioners are women, and only a quarter are men. But those men will tell you that yoga is definitely not for sissies – especially if they do the extremely aerobic Ashtanga yoga. It's a very strong work-out. But in any kind of yoga, I defy anyone to hold almost any of the standing poses for longer than a minute without breaking out into a sweat. Unlike pumping weights or running a marathon on a treadmill, yoga gives the body a complete workout, increasing endurance, building strength, stretching all the muscle groups (whilst preventing injury), and stimulating the internal organs – which is something no other workout does.

'Men often suffer from tightness particularly in the hips, hamstrings and shoulders that can lead to injury or weakness,' according to Baron Baptiste, a former coach to with the Philadelphia Eagles. 'Overtraining in any one sport can cause repetitive stress and other more serious injuries. Yoga is a full-body workout that creates both strength and flexibility. You need to have both: one without the other is a recipe for disaster.'

Many men admit to starting yoga because they have been dragged along to classes by their wives or girlfriends; other men think it might be a great way to meet a girlfriend. Increasingly, GPs are referring men to yoga classes. In my health club in Banbury, the local hospital regularly suggests the yoga classes there to men who have high blood pressure, heart or other health problems as a way of getting fitter without fear of injury. Weight-lifters are another group who are so muscle-bound that they often have very limited mobility and are directed to yoga as a way of stretching out their muscles.

My yoga teacher, Marilyn, recalls teaching a form of Ashtanga yoga at a city club in London back in 2000. 'It was bonus time and cocaine was rife but these city types used to use my classes on a Sunday morning to cure their hangovers,' she says. 'Word got around that the yoga I was doing was 'power yoga' where you sweat such a lot that you shake off your Saturday night indulgences. The studio was very hot, the guys were very competitive and when I went round the class adjusting them, I could smell the alcohol fumes on them – knew exactly what each one of them had been drinking!' So popular was Marilyn's hangover cure, that the class was always overflowing and she had to have a man like a bouncer on the door.

Back in more sedate Banbury, in soberer times, she now sees quite a lot of men who, having ignored health problems for as long as they can, get a big wake up call one day in the form of a minor heart attack or similar and start coming to yoga where, she says, they feel the benefits straight away. 'I also get quite a few of the 'worried well' who anticipate health problems and attempt to stave them off.' With a high proportion of middle aged to elderly men in some of her classes, she tries Yin yoga with them – a form of very gentle yoga performed sitting down or lying down where you hold poses for several minutes and do stretches that penetrate the deep muscle tissues which has proved very popular with both men and women of a certain age.

Of course, body-conscious gay men are very up for yoga and you can find gay yoga classes in cities like London and New York. An adjunct to this is Gay nude yoga (yep, don't let's even think of Downward Dog…) which needless to say is doing really well and which I discuss later.

So, time to try out yoga on my own family. My husband finally says he will give it a go sometime but when we have the teacher there and the mat comes out, he pleads a 'sore knee'. I have more success with my 26-year-old son who goes to the gym whenever he has the time and can do 100 press-ups as quickly as I can eat a packet of crisps. He is astonished by how difficult he finds the asanas. 'I couldn't believe that I was unable to touch my toes with straight legs,' he says. 'When I watch people doing yoga, it looks effortless and I was sure I would be able to do it, no problem.' In fact, he found it very difficult in his first lesson but absolutely got the point. 'I felt such a good stretch in the twists, and was interested in how breathing into the posture can help so much.' Like most young men, he was very strong, but very stiff in the lower back. 'He needs to use his lower back muscles, open up his chest and lengthen his neck', said his yoga teacher.

But it's still hard work getting men on mats – especially the ones who would benefit the most. Back in the day, yoga was practised exclusively by men. Nowadays, it's a brave man who unfurls his mat among all the girls who still seem to favour pink mats years after they threw away their Barbies. Oh, and the other big fear of men, I've discovered, is their flatulence issues. The journalist A.A. Gill who caught the yoga bug in Bali revealed in a recent interview: 'I plan to do it (yoga) privately at home because before yoga finds your well of serenity, it finds your canister of gas, and I couldn't do it in a room of Fulham girls'.

Unhelpful too are cult film clips like 'Inappropriate Yoga Guy' in which the star, Ogden, is clearly more interested in seducing his fit classmate Kimberly than in attaining spiritual nirvana. Ogden's antics include OM-ing too loudly, bragging about his intimacy with Sherpas in Nepal, and regularly invading Kimberly's space. When rejected, his pouting refrain is: 'Somebody didn't eat their Goji berries this morning!'

Yes, we've all come across an Ogden, so it's especially hard for men who genuinely want to do yoga rather than use it as a dating tool. Not only might they be intimidated by being perceived as an Ogden, but also they have to get past their possible embarrassment at being far less flexible than their female classmates. Stretching out muscles takes a back seat in most mens' lives and they have different problem body zones. The good news is that many of the yoga asanas are especially ideal for men. Baron Baptiste, for example, has compiled his ten best poses for men which are:

1. Forward Fold (stretches hamstrings, calves and hips; strengthens legs and knees)

2. Downward Dog (stretches feet, shoulders, hamstrings and calves; strengthens arms, legs and core)

3. Chair (stretches shoulders and chest; strengthens thighs, calves, spine and ankles)

4. Crescent Lunge (Loosens tight hips by stretching the groin; strengthens arms and legs)

5. Warrior I (stretches shoulders and hips;

strengthens upper and lower body)

6. Bridge (Stretches chest, neck, spine and hips)

7. Bow Pose (stretches hips, shoulders and thighs; strengthens back)

8. Boat Pose (strengthens abs, spine, arms and hip flexors)

9. Hero Pose (stretches knees, ankles and thighs)

10. Reclining Big Toe (stretches hips, thighs, hamstrings, groins and calves; strengthens knees)

Men in yoga also have to get past their competitive urges and inability to focus on one thing at a time, but once they do, they swear by the emotional benefits of yoga. 'It's a kind of freedom that we don't get in daily life,' says one man I spoke to. 'Many men, especially if they are business types, or aggressive sportsmen, need to learn to relax and let go. It's difficult at first but once you do it, you don't look back. It's a kind of freedom.'

So, boys, if you can get past the social, physical and emotional barriers that discourage men from practising yoga, you will benefit hugely. And no, for those of you who are more testosterone fuelled, you don't have to chant or tune into your inner girl, you can look on it as a chance to get rock-hard abs and boost your sexual prowess (but that's another story).

14

Does God believe in Yoga?

On Friday 31st August, 2007, *The Times* carried a report which caused a stir under the headline 'Vicars ban unchristian yoga for toddlers'. It outlined that a children's exercise class had been banned from two church halls because that exercise was yoga, and the vicars described yoga as unchristian. The yoga teacher, Miss Woodcock, was said to have been outraged by their ban on her 'Yum-Yum Yoga class for toddlers and mums' claiming that 'yoga is a completely non-religious activity'. She did, however, concede that 'some types of adult yoga are based on Hindu and Buddhist meditation, but it is not part of the religion and there is no dogma involved'.

Miss Woodcock, understandably, was trying to 'defuse' yoga of its spiritual connotations which appear 'unsafe' to Christians (even though one might have been tempted to ban the class for its gag-inducing title alone).

I have touched on my anxieties about the whole spiritual side of yoga but my determination to do the physical practice was only reinforced when I started to realise how anti-yoga certain Christians are. English vicars are bad enough, but try American fundamentalists.

'Satan is using Yoga to seduce the gullible', according to a loony born-again Christian on the net:

> Q: I do yoga exercises because I am fat. Is it OK?
> A: Yikes no! You cannot pretend that just doing the exercises is harmless. Yoga is entirely based upon the occult, and by joining in you honour Satan and rebel against the Lord Jesus Christ: Deu 5:7, 1Co 10: 18-23. Christ will give you all the self control and self discipline you need to reduce your weight as you get filled with His Spirit.

Oh well, that's all right then.

Many Christians believe yoga to be a 'false religion' because during the practice of yoga, the yogi is 'yoking' himself to Hindu gods. They are fond, I discovered, of quoting from 2 Corinthians 6:14: 'Be ye not unequally yoked together with unbelievers.'

'As a Christian,' says one, 'our spiritual antennae should immediately go up when we encounter a practice that uses words like 'union' or 'yoke.' The fact that these words appear frequently in the bible is overlooked...

The debate rages on. In both the UK and the US, many churches forbid yoga practice among their followers. On the other hand, confusingly, since 2005 there has been a movement called Christian Yoga and a network of Christian yoga teachers which has also spawned books like *Yoga for Christians* by Susan Bordenkircher. In fact, as long ago as 1960, a Benedictine monk called Father J.M. Dechanet published *Christian Yoga*, a respected book in which he outlines how he found in yoga a valuable approach to Christian prayer and practice – a combination so arcane at the time that it merited a feature in *Time* Magazine.

Kristy DiGeronimo is a member of Spring Branch Community Church in Virginia Beach and is allowed to use their Sunday School room for Christian yoga. What this means essentially is that she and her students do yoga poses whilst reciting the Lord's Prayer. She maintains that the ancient practice can be infused with Christianity. 'The word yoga means 'yoke', and that ties in with Christianity so well because Jesus Christ says: 'My yoke is easy and my burden is light', she argues. (I knew the word 'yoke' wasn't entirely devil speak).

She says that as a Christian, she also used to suspect yoga. 'I thought it'd be inviting some spirits in that were not the way I wanted to go.' That was until she got a shoulder injury and then 'I felt led by the Lord to take yoga and meld it with Christian principles.' At a recent class, she opened with a bible reading and prayer to the Father while sitting in the lotus yoga position.

But at another church round the corner, the Rev. Peter E. Prosser, who is both a priest at Galilee Episcopal Church in Virginia Beach and a Christian history professor at Regent University's divinity school, takes a very different view. Yoga, he says on his church's website, 'is designed to bring you into a spiritual realm of demonic powers. You cannot separate yoga from Hinduism by giving it a Christian sugar-coating. If you are in yoga (even Christian yoga), get out! Repent of being involved.' And one of his sympathisers adds: 'The body positions were designed to open up doors to demonic influence in people's lives.'

For a properly intellectual discussion of Christian attitudes to Yoga, I recommend an essay written by Dr Christine Mangala Frost, an Indian academic born a Hindu who became a Christian at the age of 22 and has been an Orthodox Christian for several years. She was brought up with yoga as her grandfather was a friend of one of founders of modern yoga, Swami Sivananda, who used to send the family his books.

She presents arguments both for and against Christians incorporating yoga into their lives based on a proper understanding of the philosophy underlying both yoga and Christianity. She has little time for the way in which, encouraged by the propaganda of Hindu missionary gurus such as Swami Vivekananda (who, in 1893, made a pilgrimage from Bombay to Chicago to spread the message to the World's Parliament of Religions), yoga has been stripped of its mystique and complexity and 'remoulded in the idiom of American schools of self-help and positive thinking and marketed as a safe and easy pathway to bliss within the grasp of all'. The employment of certain yoga techniques to promote that yoga buzz word 'self-realisation' is one of the main reasons, according to Dr Frost, why yoga might be incompatible with Christianity where the focus on self as opposed to God is considered the root of all evil.

Given that the spiritual goals of yoga are incompatible with Christianity, she asks whether there is a way a Christian can disengage from the Hindu ethos, use its techniques and still remain a committed Christian, and concludes: 'Christians undertaking yoga should be fully aware of this incompatibility but if you are well grounded in Christian thinking, prayer and Christian living, it should be possible, by the grace of God, to take what is good in yoga, and discard its alien ethos. Attempts to Christianize Yoga are commendable but may prove distracting'.

Though I don't agree with her entirely, she is certainly a voice of reason when compared with the snake-twirling fundamentalist American pastors.

But fundamentalist Christians aren't the only ones to object to the multi billion dollar yoga industry in the United States. A new controversy has burgeoned involving a small but influential group of American Hindus who have launched a 'Take Back Yoga' movement to draw attention to the deeply Hindu and Indian religious roots of yoga, which, they feel, the industry has jettisoned in order to sell yoga to the secular mainstream. The group behind the campaign, the Hindu American Foundation, does not want yoga devotees to become Hindu – it just wants the debt acknowledged. 'Hinduism has lost control of the brand', explained Dr Aseem Shukla, the foundation's co-founder.

The debate has aroused strong feelings and gone viral, with much blog and web activity devoted to asking: Who owns Yoga? And the *New York Times* recently ran a lead story on it. The new age writer and pop philosopher Dr Deepak Chopra has dismissed the objections as 'faulty history and Hindu nationalism'. In June, though, the Indian Government were prompted to register and make digital copies of drawings showing the provenance of more than 4000 yoga poses to discourage claims by entrepreneurs like Bikram Choudhury, the Indian born yoga instructor and founder of Hot yoga or Bikram yoga, from copyrighting his personal 26 yoga poses as 'Bikram Yoga'.

The images are intended to promote irrefutable evidence that Indians created the yoga asanas. 'It's like soccer and Britain,' Suneel Singh, one of India's leading yogis, told the *Guardian*, 'you have given it to the world which is wonderful and generous. But imagine other people saying that they had invented the sport. That would be annoying.'

Just one of the millions of 'Holy Wars' going on in the world I guess.

If I thought that God might be an obstacle to my yoga practice, I now have to tell you that I also feel distinctly uncomfortable about all the happy-clappy, touchy-feely, New Age industry that seems to have grown up around yoga. Look on any yoga website and the chances are that you will be linked into a whole heap of twaddle like horoscopes, crystal gazing, tarot cards, relationship advice based on moon cycles, rune stones and many other absurdities.

It is often said that yoga is a one-stop shop for mind, body and soul. And I can see that. It's certainly good for the mind and body, as I have outlined and as good science confirms. The soul? Well, that's obviously the sticking point. People talk about their yogic 'journeys', their cosmic energy, the fact that Mercury is in retrograde… what?

Writing in the online magazine, Slate, the caustic American journalist Ron Rosenbaum refers to 'the hostile New Age takeover of yoga' meaning the intolerably smug and narcissistic terms in which some yogis express themselves. 'At its best,' he writes, 'it's harmless mental self-massage. At its worst, it's the kind of thinking that blames cancer victims for their disease because they didn't 'manifest' enough positive vibes.'

He goes on to say: 'One 'manifestation' of this takeover is the shameless enlistment of yoga and elevated Eastern yogic philosophy for shamelessly material Western goals' like burning fat, de-stressing and having meaningful relationships.

If you want more examples of the mass delusion that is positive thinking, which worryingly seems to have been annexed on to large parts of the yoga industry, I urge you to read research scientist Barbara Ehrenreich's

superb and timely attack, in her book *Smile or Die,* on
the growing phenomenon of positive thinking – the
lethal kind that dismisses disturbing news and eschews
any kind of critical thinking. She herself fell victim to
the 'pink ribbon culture' when she was diagnosed with
breast cancer and bombarded with advice to positively
embrace the disease – the implication being that if she
didn't, her tumour would only grow bigger. As she says,
thereby placing a secondary burden on the cancer suf-
ferer. She survived in spite of not smiling through it
and has this to say: 'Breast cancer, I can now report, did
not make me prettier or stronger, more feminine or
spiritual. What it gave me…was a very personal, agonising encounter with an ideological force in American
culture that I had not been aware of before – one that
encourages us to deny reality, submit cheerfully to mis-
fortune, and blame only ourselves for our fate.'

Much of this stuff is just sloppy thinking and pretty
harmless but when the multi-billion 'motivational
industry' becomes involved as it has to a mind-boggling
degree in the yoga world (which I come to later), then
you have wonder. And, it's worth pointing out, the
alternative to positive thinking does not have to be
despair (which can be just as delusional), realistic
assessment is still an option. Realism is a prerequisite
not only for human survival but for all animal species.
A wild animal that isn't constantly checking out what's
behind it, won't last long.

Just to make you laugh, here is an example of the
harmless type of self-serving battiness that plagues

certain corners of the yogic world: I came across a woman called Ingrid Steimer in Canada offering a Chocolate Yoga Workshop. I quote: 'Experience a reconnection of your senses with Mother Nature's gift of chocolate as you move through a gentle series of Hatha yoga postures. You will savour the taste of a variety of organic antioxidant-rich chocolate from different parts of the world while learning the benefits of moment-to-moment mindfulness through your asana practice. Discover the wonder of nature and yoga to bring you to a new level of awareness and appreciation. Yoga teaches one to be more present, and being present in the moment adds more flavour to the moment. Yoga will allow you to savour what is being awakened through a symphony of inspiring chocolate...'

You really couldn't make it up.

15

'Corporate Karma'

What is less difficult to believe than Chakras is that yoga, in the course of a few decades, has become a multi-billion dollar industry in the West. One in ten Americans now practise yoga and it's estimated that the percentage increases by 20-25 per cent every year. Three quarters of these are women so it's perhaps not surprising that yoga merchandise and paraphernalia from Gucci sticky mats to high-end designer yoga apparel has become big business and that thousands of yogis 'see no contradiction between the spiritual aims of their discipline and the worldly symphony of ringing cash registers' in the words of *Vanity Fair* magazine.

According to the Yoga Business Academy ('We show yoga business owners like you how to increase profits using proven marketing designed specifically for yoga!') founded by Tamara Machavariani, spending on yoga products has increased by 87 per cent in the last five years. Her website asks 'Fact: 6 Billion spent annually on yoga. What's your cut?' The Academy exists to help yoga studios, yoga teachers, yoga retreats, yoga merchandise distributors to get a bigger cut of a deliciously proliferating market.

Tamara says that it will only get bigger. Her predictions include: Asia will be the next growth market; insurance companies are already paying for yoga; yoga will be prescribed by the doctor in the near future; companies looking to associate their products or services with a wellness lifestyle will turn to yoga imagery (think Worldly-Wise by Morgan Stanley). A sexy yogini, she adds, sipping a glass of wine while sitting in lotus position on the hood of a car is not out of the question if it helps sell the car.

On Asia being the next growth market, B.K.S. Iyengar was recently the star attraction at China's first ever 'yoga summit' where he was met by an enthusiastic audience of over a thousand yogis. Yoga has flourished in China in recent years in spite of China having its own indigenous systems of mind-body regimes. 'The response here (in China) has been unbelievable,' said Iyengar. 'I will not be surprised if China even overtakes India in yoga.'

A few years ago, the yoga blogs in the U.S. got wind of a talent agency for wannabe celebriyogis – yoga teachers who need effective public relations to make them into world-class brands (so yogic…) and, sure enough, the Yoga Artist Management Agency founded by Ava Taylor was born. Suddenly, yoga teachers became the new celebrity chefs, complete with television spots, events and product endorsements. 'We help teachers by managing all the nitty-gritty business details. From developing a brand identity to organizing tours, booking photo shoots and leveraging social media, we do it all', says their website.

'I can contact every yoga teacher of significance on the planet in about an hour,' boasts Ms Taylor, 31, whose agency handles bookings and strategy for 45 teachers. One of her first clients was Sadie Nardini, who describes herself as a 'Life Stylist, Ultimate Wellness Expert and Founder of Core Strength Vinyasa yoga who lives in Brooklyn, New York,' but frequently goes on the road 'to share her expertise'. One might wonder why she needs an agent with that kind of chutzpah. But here's why: Sadie aspires to become another Anthony Bourdain, the brash TV chef. 'He's the bad boy of food, and I am the black sheep of yoga,' Ms Nardini told the *New York Times*. When asked about the ethos of seeking material rewards for her spiritual endeavours, Ms Nardini explained: 'My landlord doesn't take karma'.

Ms Taylor started YAMA in 2009 after quitting her job in marketing for the cult yoga clothing company lululemon athletica, whose signature clinging 'Groove Pant' no self-respecting fashion-conscious yogini can afford to be without (at 98 dollars a pair).

But just in case you thought money-making was what Lululemon was all about, up pops its founder Chip Wilson, on his website to tell us that: 'Goal setting is a big part lululemon culture. Every employee is encouraged to set personal, health, and career goals and is given goal setting training so we can set goals that are powerful and meaningful to us.' The company also pays for management staff and other employees who have worked for the company for over a year to attend the Landmark Forum, a 'personal development' course, which draws its materials from Scientology.

Lululemon's first store was in Vancouver, Canada, but it's now absolutely massive with hundreds of stores all over Canada and the States and is currently looking for a UK site in one of London's more affluent areas. Unfortunately, for Lululemon, the wholesome brand and personal development image has been somewhat tarnished by a sensational murder case in which one female employee has been convicted of killing another in the Bethesda, Maryland Lululemon store.

Tara Stiles is typical of a new breed of rebel yoginis. A former model from Illinois, she owns Strala yoga in New York which she has built into a powerful yoga brand complete with a couple of star devotees – Jane Fonda and Deepak Chopra. Stiles, also known in the press as 'the sexy yogini', dispenses with the Sanskrit names for poses, chanting and chakras. Her yoga is pitched as another fitness regime for the body beautiful.

She has successfully outraged the conventional yoga industry. Her how-to book is entitled *Slim, Calm, Sexy*, and her short online videos have titles like 'Yoga for a Hangover' and 'Couch Yoga'. Interviewed recently in the *New York Times*, she says: 'I feel like I'm standing up for yoga. People need yoga, not another religious leader.' She refuses to pledge allegiance to one teacher, one studio or even one style of yoga. She eschews what she perceives as yoga elitism or purism, aiming instead to attract ordinary people who might be put off by chanting or talk of enlightenment. 'One of the things I like about her is her ability to make yoga accessible to people who might be scared of it or think it might be too esoteric,' Jane Fonda said of Ms Stiles.

Stiles shrugs off the criticism that is launched at her from every quarter, especially from indignant yoga bloggers. 'Who made these rules?' she asks. 'I was never invited to the party anyway – so I started my own party.'

The likes of Tara Stiles and Sadie Nardini may consider themselves the black sheep of yoga, but they have surely been eclipsed by the real bad boy of yoga, Bikram Choudhury.

In 2011 a BBC presenter Jolyon Jenkins broadcast a programme on Radio 4 wittily entitled 'Corporate Karma' in which he investigated the yoga business phenomenon. One of his main interviewees was the renowned apostate founder of 'hot yoga' whose 'Bikram Yoga' franchises have made him a mountain of money. But not content to cruise round Hollywood in one of his white Rolls Royce Silver Clouds wearing his legendary uber bling watch encrusted with diamonds, Bikram also has got himself into hot water by making some extravagant claims that cannot be verified. Here he is on what makes him so special:

'In 1959, the Beatles come to me, George Harrison come to me in Calcutta, introduced by Ravi Shankar.

In 1960, Shirley MacLaine she come to me and tell

me and say America needs someone like me, please come to Hollywood, but I didn't have any intention to leave India as I am doing very good in India. I am teaching prime minister, Indira Ghandi, a movie star in Bombay, all the businessmen. Then in 1972 I go to teach President Nixon. He has phlebitis thrombosis in left leg so they put me in the air force plane and I teach President Nixon – 7 lessons in 3 days and pain is disappear. So Nixon give me a green card gift...'

Here Jolyon says: 'The Nixon episode doesn't appear in the President's memoirs and in 1959 the Beatles didn't exist so Bikram's anecdotes may not be completely accurate...' When Jolyon then wonders whether all the glowing testimonials on Bikram's website of people being cured of pain would stand up to medical scrutiny, Bikram tells him that of course they would, that he works with the American Medical Association; that he does research with NASA and all the top universities. More claims that cannot be verified – 'Nasa could find no trace of a research programme into yoga for astronauts' comments Jolyon.

Later in the year, A *Times* journalist, Damian Whitworth, was verbally abused by Bikram and kicked out of his hotel suite whilst attempting to verify some of his more fantastic claims. He has also angered the Indian Government by attempting to claim copyright in 2002 in the 26 postures that make up the specific sequence that is Bikram yoga. The poses, argues Dr V.K. Gupta, who heads the Traditional Knowledge Digital Library in Delhi, are not his to copyright – they are in the public domain and have been so for thousands of years. The government has now started to video thousands of yoga postures and is lodging them with international patent offices to stop other opportunists like Bikram claiming they have created new types of yoga. 'Nobody should misappropriate yoga and start charging franchise money,' says Gupta.

But this is precisely what Bikram has done, and he has grown mega-rich doing it. He makes millions of dollars a day. Bikram yoga is the Starbucks of the yoga world and teachers pay him $7000 (£4250) to do his nine week training course. His followers – who reportedly include Elle Macpherson, Daniel Craig, George Clooney and Andy Murray – swear by the benefits of practising his yoga sequence in rooms heated up to 40 degrees centigrade to mimic India, but he has made as many enemies as friends throughout the yoga community. His friends acknowledge that his flamboyant wealth and vitriolic outbursts (he recently called American yoga 'a fucked up circus' and its teachers 'clowns') sit uneasily with the idea of a Yogi being a humble man of wisdom and peace for whom spiritualism is the key, rather than money. But they are extraordinarily forgiving. 'He's ostentatious in his wealth, but underneath he really cares', one of Bikram's teachers in Bristol, tells Jolyon Jenkins. Bless!

'I don't give a shit what the fuck people think about me,' he informs Damian Whitworth. 'They sick people. They are idiot people, they are stupid people. I educate them… I keep people alive for 100 years. That's my job.

That's why pope come to me (um, no he didn't).
Presidents come to me. Whole world come to me.' And
so on.

Bikram may be the most high profile yogi to have
made a fortune out of the yoga phenomenon, but he's
by no means the only one. Yogi Bhajan, the late popu-
lariser of Kundalini yoga in America, saw no conflict
between spirituality and material wealth. He amassed a
huge number of business enterprises including Akal
Security, a firm that specializes in protecting government sites, military installations, missile ranges, civil
amenities and even airports across the US.

John Friend is a case in point. Founder of the 'heart-
opening' Anusara yoga, one of the world's fastest-
growing styles of yoga, he has created various global
businesses based on Anusara schools, publishing ven-
tures, yoga-wear etc. Anusara Inc. currently makes
about £2 million a year in revenue. He is the sole stock-
holder in the company and pays himself a salary that is
just under $100,000 according to the *New York Times*.
On commercialisation, he says: 'I strongly believe that
all the downsides of commercialisation… are far out-
weighed by the potential of millions of people to
realise their divine nature.' Right.

Like other celebrity yogis, Friend has become a
brand himself, complete with book deals, fashion lines,
studio franchises and intellectual property lawsuits.
How did yoga, that centuries-old spiritual discipline
become a fitness routine that has taken the world by
storm? For anyone interested in this, I recommend a

new book by the journalist Stefanie Syman – a founder of the web magazine *Feed* – entitled: *The Subtle Body: The Story of Yoga in America.*

So, depending on your viewpoint, the proliferation of the yoga marketplace is a way of reaching out to millions more, or a necessary evil. One modest teacher I spoke to said ruefully that in the last 15 years or so, it had become much harder to practise yoga – both on and off the mat.

Conclusion

At the Yoga Show held each year in London's Olympia, I start to panic. There are hundreds of exhibitors all pushing leaflets into your hand, all wanting to sell you something or persuade you to take part in a lottery. In the first ten minutes I was: cordially invited to wash my hands in some kind of dead sea crystal salt, urged to enter the 'Meditation Tent', sold a neti pot, told I looked like I needed spiritual cleansing (by a man called Ocean who wanted to 'activate my God-code'). I also tasted natural coconut water and marvelled at its plentiful electrolytes, was offered an Ayurvedic non-surgical facelift, and got cornered into an earnest conversation with a woman about having to acknowledge the arrival of the Aquarian Age.

In amongst the madness, however, there were some inspiring yoga workshops and demonstrations, some just about affordable yoga accessories and reading material, and an opportunity for serious yogis to decide which of the many yoga training courses and workshops they wanted to attend.

Yoga has become huge – and the word 'yoga' is now an umbrella term that seems to cover everything from staring into Mystic Meg's crystal ball to serious mental and physical disciplines. The only sensible way forward is to work out what you personally want from it and are prepared to give to it.

For those who are lost, stressed, unhappy, unfocussed, addicted – for people looking for answers and a way to fill the void in their lives – yoga is manifestly transformational. For many people, yoga has replaced family, replaced the church, and replaced everything that is lacking in their lives. It's confessional, it's safe, it's non-exclusive and it's non-judgemental. There is a wide and welcoming global yoga community and you, whoever you are and whatever your background is, can belong. This is the message.

Yoga is practised, not just in village halls or shiny urban studios, but everywhere. It is widely used in the workplace, as therapy for addicts and troubled teenagers, even for the purpose of conflict resolution. It can't be long before we watch politicians launch into downward dogs at political summits. In boardrooms from Manhattan to Manila, the mantra 'let's do lunch' is being replaced by 'let's do yoga'.

I started off cynical and I have ended up less cynical. I am still doubtful about the rapidly commercialising yoga industry, the aggressively un-yogic 'yoga entrepreneurs', about the inflated egos of yoga teacher-gods, about the dumbing down of the practice to suit the western notion of 'a wellness lifestyle', about overpriced designer togs and sticky mats, and, most of all, about the stream-of-drivel 'spiritual industry' that attends this quiet, ancient esoteric practice of yore. But, I am not cynical about the physical practice of yoga itself which, much to my surprise, I have found challenging but fulfilling as well as mentally restful. Oh, ok, healing if you must. And I have seen for myself the transformation it has brought about in others. In the words of B.K.S. Iyengar, 'Words cannot covey the value of yoga – it has to be experienced.'

Appendix I

Choose Your Own Style of Yoga

There are so many styles of yoga being practised today globally, especially in the United States (where the latest estimates put the number of people practising yoga at a staggering 20 million, and the possible number of styles of yoga at around 280) that it can be completely bewildering, and very difficult to decide which style to go for. Let me just run a few of them by you so you get the picture:

Hatha, Ashtanga, Iyengar, Kundalini, Bikram, Viniyoga, Anusara, Jivamukti, Kripalu, Sivananda – and so on.

All of these and many others are based on the same physical poses, but some are more challenging and faster – like Ashtanga – and others place more emphasis on the spiritual side of yoga, or breathing practice. Some may not be appropriate for people with certain medical problems. Certain teachers and yogis are associated with certain styles. For example, Bikram yoga, which is practised in 38 degree heat, was pioneered by Bikram Choudhury.

It might be helpful here to attempt a brief description of the more popular styles, although many yoga teachers incorporate different influences into their teaching, and not all yoga classes fall neatly into one particular style.

Hatha Yoga:

Perhaps the most common term for yoga in the west. It's a generic term that can encompass many of the physical types of yoga and the traditional asanas. If a class is described as Hatha, it is likely to be quite gentle, slow-paced and a good introduction to the poses.

The word 'Hatha' is a compound of the words 'ha' and 'tha' meaning sun and moon and is associated with the Yogi Swatmarama, a sage of 15th century India, who compiled the Hatha yoga Pradipika text, which was in turn derived from older texts. The word itself actually means 'forceful' and is taken to refer to a strong physical practice, purifying the body in preparation for higher meditation.

Ashtanga (Power) Yoga:

Ashtanga means 'eight limbs' in Sanskrit and is a fast paced, intensely aerobic style of yoga in which a set series of poses, usually Sun Salutations, are performed, often in the same order. Each pose flows into the next one by means of Vinyasa (breath-synchronised) movement and is physically demanding. The purpose of Vinyasa is for internal cleansing. Synchronizing breathing and movement in the asanas heats the blood, cleaning and thinning it so that it circulates more freely relieving joint pain and removing toxins from the internal organs. The sweat generated then carries these impurities out of the body.

Ashtanga was founded by K. Pattabhi Jois (1915-2009) and has become global. The original Ashtanga Institute is in Mysore, India.

Iyengar Yoga:
Based on the teachings of the yogi B.K.S. Iyengar, this style of practice is most concerned with correct bodily alignment – meaning the precise way your body should be positioned in each asana in order to obtain maximum benefit and avoid injury. These aligned poses are then held for a minute or two. Iyengar practice encourages the use of props such as blocks and straps as aids in performing the poses. Like Ashtanga, it is also based on the traditional eight limbs of yoga and is a form of Hatha yoga.

Iyengar yoga is often used as therapy on patients with physical problems because it assists in the manipulation of inflexible or injured areas. Iyengar himself worked with patients who had suffered myocardial infarctions. There are well documented studies of the benefits of Iyengar yoga on people with osteoarthritis, chronic backache, immunodeficiency, high blood pressure, insomnia, depression and menopausal symptoms.

Iyengar is taught around the world and there are several institutes in both the UK and the US. The original one is the Ramamani Iyengar Institute in Pune,

India, established by B.K.S. Iyengar in memory of his wife.

Bikram Yoga:

Or hot yoga, pioneered by Bikram Choudhury, who introduced his system in the U.S. in 1971. It is practised in a very hot room (105 degrees) which encourages loosening of tight muscles and profuse sweating which is thought to be cleansing. The Bikram method is a set series of 26 poses but not every class uses this. Each class is 90 minutes long, 45 minutes of standing poses and 45 minutes of floor postures. The HQ is The Bikram Yoga College of India in Los Angeles and there are now thousands of certified Bikram teachers throughout the U.S. and the U.K.

Kundalini Yoga:

The emphasis is on the breath in conjunction with physical movement with the purpose of freeing energy (prana) in the lower body and allowing it to move upwards. The primary objective is 'to awaken the full potential of human awareness in each individual'. The 'Breath of Fire', a pranayama exercise characterised by rapid and rhythmic exhalations, is the hallmark of a Kundalini class, which typically will begin with chanting and ends with singing. In-between are asanas, pranayama and meditation (or kriya). Kundalini yoga was founded in the U.S. in 1969 by Yogi Bhajan and there is a Kundalini Research Institute and International Training Center in New Mexico.

Viniyoga:

Based on personalised programs for each student devised by an experienced teacher or guru, based on factors such as age and physical condition. T.K.V. Desikachar is the world's foremost Viniyoga authority, while Gary Kraftsow, founder of the American Viniyoga Institute in 1999, is the most prominent American proponent of this method. Depending on individual need, a class could include asana, pranayama, chanting and meditation. It is usually a relatively gentle experience.

Sivananda Yoga:

Based on five principles: 1. Proper exercise (focusing on 12 particular asanas); 2. Proper breathing (Pranayama); 3. Proper Relaxation (Savasana); 4. Proper diet (Vegetarian); 5. Positive thinking and meditation. Based on the teachings of Swami Sivananda, it is more of a spiritual practice than exercise. Each class focuses on the practice of 12 core poses plus chanting, pranayama, meditation and relaxation.

The first Sivananda Yoga Center was founded in 1959 by Swami Vishnu-Devananda and there are now many locations and ashram retreats worldwide.

Yin Yoga:

All the poses are lying down or sitting down and are held for several minutes at a time. Yin yoga targets not the muscles, but the connective tissue, specifically ligaments and tendons in the joints and spine. Over time

yin yoga can lengthen these tissues increasing mobility. Yin yoga is a slow but deep practice which has both
physical and mental benefits. It is suitable for all levels
of students and is a perfect complement to the more
dynamic (yang) styles of yoga which concentrate on
stretching and contracting muscles. Excellent for the
hips, pelvis and lower spine. Yin yoga has been popu-
larized in the West by Paul Grilley and Sarah Powers.

Ansura Yoga:
Known as 'going with the flow' yoga. John Friend
founded Anusara yoga after many years of practising
and teaching Iyengar yoga. The word 'Anusara' means
'flowing with grace' and in class students are encouraged to connect with their divine nature as they apply
the five universal principles of alignment. A combo of
the physical and spiritual.

Jivamukti Yoga:
Challenging asana sequences along with Sanskrit
chanting, music and meditation. The name 'Jivamukti'
means 'liberation while living'. Sharon Gannon and
David Life founded Jivamukti yoga in 1984, choosing
the name to remind students that the ultimate aim of
the practice is enlightenment. One of the main principles of Jivamukti is non-harming and classes often
explore the link between yoga and political activism in
the areas of the environment, animal rights and veg-
anism.

*

Kripalu Yoga:
Swami Kripalu (1913-1981) was a Kundalini yoga master who taught that all the world's wisdom stems from a single universal truth which each of us can experience directly and in our own way through yoga, pranayama and meditation. Classes vary widely but students are encouraged to do what is right for their bodies and state of mind.

Then there is *Restorative Yoga* in which props are used to support the body and you hold the positions for a longer time to open up the body through passive stretching. This is wonderful for anybody who has been ill or just needs a healing practice. Restorative yoga helps to trigger the parasympathetic nervous system known as the PNS. The PNS is responsible for balancing the body and bringing it back into equilibrium.

These are the main styles of traditional yoga though you will find many others, especially in the U.S. where they are often associated with particular teachers in particular locations.* Not all yoga classes fall neatly into one particular style, though. Some are deliberately eclectic, drawing from several schools and that the only way to discover which style is appropriate for you is to try out a few and see which 'resonates with your heart' as one yoga journalist puts it. Every day a 'new' yoga style seems to emerge with people experimenting with elements of other practices such as martial arts, pilates, dance and fitness routines. The fusion of these new ele-

ments with more traditional yoga is designed to be
accessible and appealing but of course only some of
them catch on, and some are designed to target specific parts of the population: like Christian yoga. Recently
there has been a lot of press about Naked yoga (yep)
Gay Naked yoga (yes, really), Laughter yoga, and even
more alarmingly Anti-gravity yoga in which poses are
done whilst swinging above the ground in a silk
hammock.

---

* Baptiste Power Vinyasa yoga (Baron Baptiste); Forrest yoga (Ana
Forrest); Insight yoga (Sarah & Ty Powers); Integral yoga (Swami
Satchidananda); Ishta yoga (Alan Finger); Om yoga (Cyndi Lee); Parayoga
(Rod Stryker); Prana Flow yoga (Shiva Rea); Prajna yoga (Tias & Surya
Little); Purna yoga (Aadil & Mirra Palkhivala); Svaroopa yoga (Rama
Berch); Triyoga (Kali Ray); YogaFit (Beth Shaw); Moksha Hot yoga (Ted
Grant & Jessica Robertson).

Appendix II

Yoga Blogs

One of the reasons yoga seems to be taking over the world is even if they're not doing it, everybody seems to be talking about it. There are thousands of yoga bloggers all over the world (but especially in America). Some are political and try to set the agenda for the big yoga questions of the day; some are merely informative, some are devoted to yoga news and events, some are teachers trying to connect with students, some are individuals giving progress reports on their practice, some are satirical and some are inspirational. Almost all of them give lists of other blogs to follow and just a superficial surf of the net will demonstrate that you could spend the rest of your life and beyond reading about yoga thanks to all the committed bloggers who just can't stop chatting about it.

I think one of the reasons for this is that the kind of people who are attracted to yoga are believers in the building and maintaining of communities, and I have to say that the online yoga community is pretty damn impressive. The problem will always be too much information, never too little.

Personally, I started to look at a few blogs when my interest in yoga began, mostly for practical information on types of yoga, what to expect at a class, yoga poses and so on. If there's an asana that bugs you because you can't do it, there's sure to be someone on line who either shares your pain, or talks you through another way to tackle it. If you are worried because your t-shirt rides up to expose your flabby stomach, someone is sure to guide you to the right apparel that stays put even when you don't.

Blogs are a huge resource but it takes time and patience to find the ones you can relate to. There's a vast amount of self-indulgent dross out there too. Who cares if Sophie was too hung-over this morning to get on the mat or that Ben finds the pigeon pose hurts his hips? Blogs like this remind me of the craze for five year diaries we kept at school, every page of which was utterly banal – Cabbage for lunch (again), B+ in French test (!!), Pamela is a bitch, my hair needs washing, etc. etc. – nothing much there to delight and inspire future generations I fear.

One of the most enduring and popular blogs in the U.S. is YogaDork – so much so that the *New York Times* recently sought to interview the shy and retiring name behind the much-loved blog. This turns out to be Jennilyn Carson, a twenty-eight year old Jersey girl who lives in East Harlem, works in a psychotherapist's office and teaches yoga. Ms Carson's blog is written in an intelligent, ironic style and mixes pop culture with yoga issues. On the serious side, she reports on and initiates debate on whether yoga instructors should be licensed and the high cost of teacher training. She trains a half-humorous, half critical eye on the industry, labelling buyers of the costly lululemon yoga apparel as 'lul-ulemmings' and tabloid photographers who stalk yoga studios for celebrity sightings as 'yogarazzi'.

She is one of a growing number of yogis who take their yoga seriously, but bring a light, sceptical tone to their blogs. This strikes a welcome contrast with all the deathly serious ones which play new age music and throw out spiritual karma like confetti.

Others include Roseanne Harvey, the main voice behind the blog 'it's all yoga, baby', who is famously anti-consumerist and highly cynical about the increasing commercialisation of yoga, notably the rock-star status of certain yoga teachers, expensive class fees and designer yoga apparel and accessories; Neal Pollack of Nealpollack.com (subtitled The Hot Jew of the Yoga Generation), a journalist whose latest book is *Stretch: The Unlikely Making of a Yoga Dude*; Erica Rodefer, a former online editor for *Yoga Journal*, who writes as a 'spoiled yogi' at spoiledyogi.blogspot.com; Beth Lapides who claims she is 'putting the om into comedy', and my favourite of all them – YogaDawg.

YogaDawg, needless to say is a dog yogi (Sri sri swami baba guru YogaDawg) with his own biography, two disciples (MadDawg and HotDawg) and author of the seminal yoga guide *My Third Eye Itches*. YogaDawg (author unknown – to me, anyhow) confounds the yoga community's tendency to take itself seriously, though I notice that it almost always appears on everyone else's blog list – and has won many awards.

YogaDawg makes scurrilous comments on every aspect of yoga life. Here he is on yoga blogs: 'The yoga blog is the spiritual heart of yoga in the internet age. It is where yogis can yammer about the poses they did in class, be loquacious with their spiritual insights, and dissect and chart their inner and outer progress... a place to write profound dissertations on the colour of their mat, what they had for breakfast, who was in their class and whether their yoga teacher is hot or not...'

That said, there are some really good yoga blogs, especially in the U.S., and they make a colourful addition to the sum our yoga knowledge and experience. Quite often, bloggers even lead the way in breaking news and mainstream media follow their lead. Probably, from the purely practical point of view, the many blogs written by yoga teachers handing out helpful advice and sharing their expertise are the most useful.

Possibly my best find on the net was a blog entitled 'A Skeptic's thoughts about life...and yoga'. This blogger's profile reads: 'A moody intellectual with habitual pessimistic, dismissive, cynical views of self and the world was recently transformed by her yoga practice into a grateful, accepting, appreciative, hopeful and ultimately a much happier person, all within a few short months. The intellectual part of her is still trying to figure out how this magic happened.' Couldn't have put it better myself.

Appendix III

Kitcheree Recipe

---

1 Cup Mung Beans
1 Cup Basmati Rice
9 Cups Water
6-7 Cups assorted Vegetables

Masala Mixture:
¼ Cup Ghee or olive oil
4-5 Cloves of fresh Garlic, crushed in a press
2 Onions, Chopped
1 finger fresh Ginger root, peeled and minced
1 1/2 Tsp Turmeric
1 1/2 Tsp Cumin powder
3/4 Tsp Ground Coriander seed
Seeds of 5 Green Cardamom Pods (or 3/4 tsp powder)
1 Tsp Black Pepper
½ Tsp Crushed Red Chillies (more if you like spicy OR omit completely if you don't like it hot)
1 – 1 1/2 Tbsp Sea Salt

Method:
Add salt to water in a large stew pot and bring water to

a light boil.

Wash Mung beans, carefully removing any tiny stones.

Rinse Basmati Rice at least three times to remove starch.

Set mung beans and rice aside.

Chop assorted vegetables.

(Prepare the Masala Mixture while waiting for water to boil)

Heat Ghee (or Oil) in a large frying pan (preferably cast iron.)

Add garlic (using press), chopped onions, and Ginger and sauté under a medium flame. When Onions, Garlic and Ginger are translucent, add Turmeric, Cumin, Coriander, Cardamom, Crushed Chillies and Black Pepper; mix well.

When all spices are absorbed turn off flame and let sit for 5 min, covered.

(When water begins to boil)

Add mung beans to boiling water.

Reduce flame to simmering and cover and boil until the beans start to soften and open, (15-20 min.)

Add Masala Mixture to water with mung beans and vegetables.

Simmer for 20-30 minutes until soupy.

Add rice and cook an additional 15-20 min until rice is absorbed.

Shut off and let set 15-20 min.